T0190232

The Business of Geriatrics

Michael Wasserman

The Business of Geriatrics

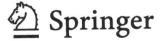 Springer

Michael Wasserman
Woodland Hills, California
USA

ISBN 978-3-319-28544-3   ISBN 978-3-319-28546-7   (eBook)
DOI 10.1007/978-3-319-28546-7

Library of Congress Control Number: 2016935192

Springer Cham Heidelberg New York Dordrecht London
© Springer International Publishing Switzerland 2016
This work is subject to copyright. All rights are reserved by the Publisher, whether the whole or part of the material is concerned, specifically the rights of translation, reprinting, reuse of illustrations, recitation, broadcasting, reproduction on microfilms or in any other physical way, and transmission or information storage and retrieval, electronic adaptation, computer software, or by similar or dissimilar methodology now known or hereafter developed.
The use of general descriptive names, registered names, trademarks, service marks, etc. in this publication does not imply, even in the absence of a specific statement, that such names are exempt from the relevant protective laws and regulations and therefore free for general use.
The publisher, the authors and the editors are safe to assume that the advice and information in this book are believed to be true and accurate at the date of publication. Neither the publisher nor the authors or the editors give a warranty, express or implied, with respect to the material contained herein or for any errors or omissions that may have been made.

Printed on acid-free paper

Springer International Publishing AG Switzerland is part of Springer Science+Business Media (www.springer.com)

Preface

It was the fall of 2000 and I was driving past the Cherry Creek Reservoir on my way home from work when I got the call from my colleague, Dr. Don Murphy. He said, "Mike, I'm going to take over my clinic downtown and try to make a go at fee-for-service Medicare. I don't know what you want to do with your clinic in Aurora but if you're interested we can do this together." I drove home, spoke to my wife, spent all evening contemplating my future, and the next morning I gave notice to resign my position as president of GeriMed of America. GeriMed was a geriatric medical management company in Denver, Colorado. I had moved to Denver just 6 years earlier and had worked my way up the ladder to the position I thought would be the pinnacle of my career. In many ways, my decision would move me down the ladder several rungs. I had never started a business from scratch. Not only was there no job security, but I would be putting my families net worth at risk. Nevertheless, on January 1, 2001, Senior Care of Colorado opened for business. Almost 10 years later, on December 1, 2010, we sold Senior Care of Colorado to IPC, The Hospitalist Company, and *I was in the position of never having to work again if I didn't want to.*

The major reason that we are even discussing the business of geriatrics is the demographic tsunami known as the baby boom. Our society has never before seen this type of growth in the older adult population. Fifty years ago, nursing homes were places that no one wanted to live in. Assisted living facilities and group homes were hardly a blip on our radar. People spent weeks in the hospital and weren't whisked away to skilled nursing facilities after three days. Alzheimer's disease wasn't even in our vocabulary. We called it senility. The pharmaceutical industry was just getting started. Pacemakers had just come on the market, and coronary bypass surgery was in its infancy. There were no schools of gerontology and no departments of geriatric medicine.

I have been told many times over the years that practicing geriatrics is not synonymous with financial success. What has surprised me is how many people continue to tell me this. Not only did I practice geriatrics for many years, but I have also been part of organizations that have demonstrated that one can make a very good living doing so. I have tried various ways of sharing my knowledge and experience with others so that they might achieve the same personal and financial success. The most common refrain as to why physicians aren't interested in learning how to do this is that they're too busy and working too hard with little financial reward! The other, and perhaps more challenging, response has to do with the need for individuals to learn from their own mistakes. Having made my share of mistakes, I decided that a book could be a useful way of helping others achieve their goals.

It is my hope that through this book I can share what I have learned over the past 25 years. Many of us, and physicians in particular, are experiential learners. I have many stories about key moments along the way that I believe can help others understand what it takes to make geriatrics a successful business model. With that said, this book is not just for someone interested in a private geriatrics practice. The principles that I will espouse, and the experiences that I will share, are pertinent to many healthcare practice settings, from academic programs to large group practices.

It's often said that physicians don't make good businessmen. This may seem like a good excuse, but it doesn't really make sense. If physicians are smart enough to take care of complex frail elderly patients and their families, they should be able to learn to navigate the complexities of running a successful business. *They just have to want to do it.* There are many changes going on today in the healthcare marketplace, and the alternatives to private practice may or may not be appealing. Physicians tend to be very independent-minded people, and market forces are pushing them in a direction that is anathema to professionals who don't like being told what to do. *This book will give the interested reader the tools by which to retake control over their professional well-being.*

Physicians spend the first 2 years of medical school taking courses on anatomy, biochemistry, physiology, cell biology, etc. These classes become building blocks on the way to becoming clinicians. They do not encounter building blocks that will enable them to become managers or businessmen. Perhaps it shouldn't be surprising that physicians and other healthcare professionals don't have a good foundation or understanding of business principles. That is not all, though. There are plenty of people in healthcare who have gone to business school, and there are a growing number of physicians who have gone on to get an MBA. All we need to do is look around and see the state of our healthcare system today in order to determine that our business school programs may not be teaching the right principles. This appears to be the conundrum. While espousing that we teach business principles to physicians, at the same time I am saying that traditional business education may not be sufficient to be successful in today's healthcare marketplace. Businesses are only now beginning to understand the impact of the baby boom. As clinicians with expertise in geriatrics, we have a unique knowledge regarding this rapidly growing population. Societies around the world are grappling with the reality of the exploding expenditures required to care for older adults. *The solution may very well be in the intersection of our knowledge of medicine, business, and the aging of our society.*

Melding all of this together is where being an experiential learner matters the most. I hope that this book will provide the building blocks necessary to allow doctors and others in the healthcare arena realize that it is possible to provide high-quality care and excellent service while achieving financial viability. Caring for older adults often leads us to dealing with highly complex issues that often appear to have no solutions. Through education and experience, we are able to handle many of the challenges we face on a daily basis. The business side of the care we deliver should be no different. *What is most important is our desire to succeed and our willingness to learn the skills necessary to achieve our goals.*

Woodland Hills, CA, USA   Michael Wasserman, MD

Contents

A Geriatrician's Success Story

I am very fortunate to have been able to do something I love for the past 30 years. Almost everyone I know in the field of geriatrics can say the same thing. One generally doesn't decide to spend their days caring for older adults if they don't love it. Even as a child I gravitated to hanging out around the older people at family get-togethers. I had a very close and loving relationship with my grandparents. Ironically, when I entered medical school I wanted to become a pediatrician. It was during a third year surgical rotation that my desire to spend the rest of my career caring for older people became clear. When an elderly patient apologized for yelling at me when I woke her up early for morning rounds, I genuinely felt that she had every right to complain. The fact of the matter was that she was the patient. My mission wasn't to disturb her but to make her feel better. Older people often have a multitude of health-related problems. Complaints come with the territory. At the same time, they also have a wealth of experiences to share. My decision to become a geriatrician was an easy one. In fact, my internal medicine residency at Cedars-Sinai Medical Center became a de facto geriatric residency as I viewed every old person as an opportunity to learn more about geriatric medicine. Physicians are lifelong learners, and once I knew the direction I wanted to go in, I did everything I could to become more knowledgeable about the field of geriatric medicine.

1.1 Geriatric Fellowship

The first geriatric fellowship program in the United States was established in 1966.[1] While there weren't a lot of geriatricians around in 1988, the number was just starting to grow. I was accepted into a 2-year geriatric fellowship at UCLA. I didn't fully realize that my introduction into the business of geriatrics was already beginning.

---

[1] JK Brubaker, The Birth of a New Specialty: Geriatrics. *The Journal of Lancaster General Hospital* • Fall 2008 • Vol. 3 – No. 3.

© Springer International Publishing Switzerland 2016
M. Wasserman, *The Business of Geriatrics*, DOI 10.1007/978-3-319-28546-7_1

With a wife, daughter, and a new home, I was already moonlighting regularly at Kaiser-Permanente in Woodland Hills, California. Six months into my fellowship, I was given the opportunity to start an outpatient geriatric clinic at Kaiser. After considerable thought, I decided to move in a different direction than academic medicine. I was already feeling the drive to find a way to advance the cause of geriatric medicine in the marketplace. I let the fellowship director know of my plan to finish the fellowship after 1 year (ironically, the standard geriatric fellowship today is 1 year) and to join Kaiser-Permanente in Woodland Hills, California. The majority of the faculty at UCLA were very supportive of my opportunity.

Making the decision to leave my fellowship a year early was not easy. When I began the program, I was still considering a life in academic medicine. Clinical research and teaching interested me, but I also felt driven to make a difference. The question that I had to pose to myself at the time was whether I could make more of a difference by staying the course and taking the academic route or jumping into the healthcare marketplace and trying to assert my influence there. I loved caring for patients, and I already enjoyed teaching medical students and residents about geriatrics, but I saw the paucity of geriatricians in practice and felt that there was an opportunity to change that.

1.2   My First Job

I joined Kaiser in July of 1989 and began my journey in the healthcare world as a geriatrician. Developing an outpatient geriatric consult clinic became an opportunity to gain leadership and management skills. I also realized that wasn't enough and that I still wanted to make more of a difference. That drive led me to develop new programs and to try to influence the Kaiser model of care. It also gave me further opportunities to learn both the art of negotiation and to experience the hand-to-hand combat that is often necessary to obtain resources in an enclosed healthcare system. When I started working at Kaiser, I was given a regular panel of patients, though I had negotiated to have time carved out for developing a geriatric clinic. Over the next 5 years, my geriatric clinic time grew, and I also began spending time out in the field in nursing facilities.

Opportunities kept presenting themselves. It didn't hurt that as a geriatrician I felt that acute hospitals were often the worst place for a frail elder to be, so I volunteered to become the physician advisor to the hospital discharge planners and helped our hospital achieve some of the lowest hospital utilization numbers in the entire Kaiser system. This led to opportunities to consult with other Kaiser locations, where I had the opportunity to share my insight and approach. I finally ended up on a regional TQM (total quality management) project that looked at variation in hospital utilization throughout the region.

In the spring of 1994, I was named the cochief of the San Fernando Valley Department of Continuing Care and delivered a presentation at the Annual Meeting of the American Geriatrics Society on "Geriatrician's Roles in HMOs." It was at this meeting that I met Dr. Jim Riopelle, who told me about his company, GeriMed of America, and how it was going to transform the care of older people in the United States. Somehow, I knew that there was a big difference between being a geriatrician in a large healthcare organization and being one in a company whose sole purpose was delivering high-quality geriatric medical care. A few months later, I moved my family to Aurora, Colorado, and opened up GeriMed's flagship MedWise™ Center at The Medical Center of Aurora. Over the next few years, I learned a lot. I learned how to be a geriatrician throughout the entire continuum of care. Not only did this include an outpatient office practice, with hospital rounds being an integral part of the practice at the time, but working in geropsychiatry facilities, skilled and custodial nursing homes, assisted living facilities and performing house calls. Because GeriMed was a management company that managed hospital-based senior clinics, I learned the politics of hospital systems. Since the state of Colorado had a corporate practice of medicine law, we needed to have a physician corporation, and I was exposed to the challenges of a group of physicians trying to be organized.

1.3   Moving Up the Ladder

In 1998, I became President of GeriMed and was involved in negotiating the acquisition of a group of clinics in Orlando Florida. When the dust settled, we had set up and developed a number of geriatric clinics throughout central Florida. These clinics operated under the MedWise™ Philosophy of Care and followed guidelines that I helped incorporate into the American Geriatrics Society's position statement on ambulatory geriatric clinical care and services.[2, 3] Over the next 3 years, I commuted weekly between Denver and Florida. I learned a lot about the managed care industry and also began to understand the wide array of market forces affecting clinicians endeavoring to care for older adults. I became more knowledgeable about operating a medical practice and running a company. The Florida operation was a successful "full-risk" venture. During this time, there were myriad changes in the Denver market and for a number of reasons, GeriMed's attempt to operate a practice that was also at "full-risk" did not succeed (more on the lessons from this later). It was at this point, as President of GeriMed, that I was faced with the choice of closing our Denver clinics and moving to Florida. In this setting, I received that fateful phone call from Don Murphy, and I chose to embark in a new direction. Senior Care of Colorado, PC, was born, and I entered a new chapter in my career.

---

[2] Continuum: The MedWise™ Center – An Innovation in Primary Care Geriatrics, January–February 1998.

[3] Annals of Long-Term Care: "The AGS Position Statement on Ambulatory Geriatric Clinical Care and Services: A Call to Arms for Geriatricians," January 2001.

1.4   Going into Private Practice

The decision to acquire GeriMed's Denver assets and form Senior Care of Colorado
was made rather quickly. I had to learn how to start a business in a very short period
of time. Developing a business plan, borrowing money from a bank, finding a payroll service, and setting up billing and collection processes all had to happen quickly.
When I look back, the next 10 years were a whirlwind. We experienced many highs
and lows. What began as a small practice with 6 physicians and 2 physician assistants morphed into a rather large small business with nearly 70 clinicians and a total
of over 160 employees. In December of 2010, in another experience that served to
add to my business knowledge base, we sold Senior Care of Colorado to IPC, The
Hospitalist Company. I no longer had to work for a living if I didn't want to.

1.5   Doing What's Important

From a personal perspective, selling my business and being in a position to not have
to work was freeing. I actually spent a year and a half working solely as a clinician
before moving to California for personal reasons. Ironically, moving back to
California led my wife and I to become caregivers to my father-in-law in what
turned out to be the last year and a half of his life. Experiencing our healthcare system from the perspective of a caregiver and family member galvanized my resolve
to share my experiences with others. I was appointed to the Board of Directors of
two charitable organizations whose focus is to promote positive views of aging. I
volunteered to teach medical students how to interact with the patients. I made a
point of continuing to attend the annual American Geriatrics Society meetings. It
was here that I continued to hear the refrain that it was impossible to deliver quality
geriatric care and be financially viable at the same time. As a living example that
this is not the case, this book became the next step in my journey.

Why Geriatric Medicine Matters

Physicians typically decry the use of anecdotes. At a certain point, however, don't enough anecdotes become a case series? Being a geriatrician is not just a job; it is a way of life. For many of us, it is a calling, just like being a physician often used to be. I decided to become a geriatrician when I was a third year medical student in 1983. Since that time, I have approached my lifelong learning as a physician with the mindset of a geriatrician. Before we start delving into the business aspect of geriatrics, I'm going to address the issue of why the geriatric medical approach to care matters. In order to understand how geriatrics fits into today's complex healthcare marketplace, it is important to look at geriatrics from the perspective of a clinician, with real-life examples of situations that describe how most of us approach the care of our patients.

Even as an intern, the principles that I still hold dear today mattered to me. It was 1985, and I was doing my emergency medicine rotation in the emergency room of a private hospital. An elderly nursing home resident was brought in by the paramedics. She was in respiratory arrest and was quickly intubated. As I read through the records that had been sent by the nursing home, it immediately became apparent to me that this woman most likely had a quality of life that most people would find to be poor. She had a history of dementia and spent all of her time in bed. She was not communicative. Yet here she was, in the emergency room of a private hospital on a ventilator. This troubled me, so I looked at her chart and found the phone number of her son, who had medical power of attorney. I called him and asked a question that I have asked many thousands of times over the past 30 years: "What would your mom tell us about her wishes if she were capable of doing so?"

The answer is probably not surprising to most readers of this book. In fact, over the past 30 years, the typical answer that I receive from loved ones of demented individuals living in nursing homes is "she'd want us to shoot her." Back then, as I still do today, I told this woman's son that we could not shoot his mom but that we could respect her wishes. We did not have to use everything that medical science had available to keep her alive. In fact, we could focus on her comfort. The patient's

© Springer International Publishing Switzerland 2016
M. Wasserman, *The Business of Geriatrics*, DOI 10.1007/978-3-319-28546-7_2

son was quite relieved to hear this and we proceeded to take this woman off the ventilator. She was moved to a regular hospital unit to be kept comfortable and died shortly thereafter.

2.1   Basic Tenets of Geriatric Medicine

One of the standard tenets of geriatric medicine is to respect the dignity and autonomy of our patients. The issues of sustaining life are very complex in younger people who do not have a lifetime behind them. However, in older adults, the thought of suffering with poor quality of life is anathema to most people. With that said, it should be made clear that over the years I have had a handful of patients who had clear wishes to prolong their lives at whatever cost. I have always respected those wishes as well. Nevertheless, if we take the time to determine the wishes of our patients, we will often find that these wishes don't always correspond to the treatment of a specific disease. *It is incumbent upon us as clinicians to understand what makes our patients tick and to do everything in our power to respect those wishes.*

One may look at this example and recognize the concept of palliative care. It is interesting that an entire new specialty has developed in recent years to approach an issue that geriatricians have been addressing for many years. There is actually a business reason for this. Historically, we have not made a good business case for our approach to care. It is not surprising. The palliative approach to care generally limits the use of hospitalization, procedures, and medications. From a practical perspective, these are the key economic drivers of our healthcare system. As the overall costs of the Medicare program have exploded, the growing financial pressure from what may be considered the traditional approach to care has forced our society to look at alternatives. For a number of reasons, the market did not look at geriatric medicine as a solution but has begun to embrace palliative care. A lot of money has been poured into developing palliative care as a specialty, and ironically, as this funding has begun to dry up, the field of palliative care has begun to struggle with the same business issues that geriatricians have faced. *Nevertheless, it is important to recognize that palliative care is an important facet of the geriatric approach to care.*

2.2   My Grandfather and the Healthcare System

My next case study involved my grandfather. He was in his 80s at the time and had recently been in a motor vehicle accident. Being the driver, his chest wall had hit the steering wheel, and for 2 weeks he had ongoing problems with chest pain. Not surprisingly, going to a private hospital well known for its cardiac care, he ended up in the cardiac intensive care unit. It wasn't long before he was sedated and on multiple medications. He was also restrained. Walking into my grandfather's hospital room, I immediately knew that the situation was not right. There were many things in his history that didn't add up. Moreover, as a geriatrician, I was very concerned that he was now delirious and no matter what else happened was being put at significant risk for numerous iatrogenic complications. My grandfather was a very proud and independent man. It was immediately apparent to me that his treatment was not conducive to his wishes. I spoke to the cardiologists and told them to stop everything that they were doing. They told me that my grandfather would die if they did that. I told them that if he were to die, he would not want it to be this way. I also told them that I'd be willing to take the chance that he wouldn't die. He went home 3 days later. *Oftentimes in geriatrics, doing less is better for the patient.*

I have many thousands of stories like this, but I'm going to share one more. For many years while I was in practice in Denver, I cared for a delightful husband and wife. The husband was diagnosed with prostate cancer and treated with antihormonal therapy. Shortly after the wife passed away, the man was hospitalized with pneumonia. When I saw him for his post-discharge visit in my office, I realized that his overall condition had declined significantly. He was discernibly weaker and the essential tremor that he'd had for many years had worsened. Viewing this man through the eyes of a geriatrician, it all became clear. *We were killing this 88-year-old man's prostate cancer, and we were also killing him at the same time.*

2.3 Doing the Right Thing

Taking testosterone away from a man causes many deleterious effects, muscle weakness certainly being one of them. His testosterone level was zero, as was his PSA. I called his urologist and told him that I was planning to discontinue his antihormonal treatment and actually put him on testosterone for the time being. One can easily imagine the response of the urologist! He literally became apoplectic. After he calmed down, I asked him what level of PSA needed to occur before one typically saw metastases to the bone. I knew the answer but wanted him to tell me. It was a PSA of 30. I made him a deal. I told him that if my patient's PSA ever got close to 30, we would put him back on his treatment. Why did I do this? Over the course of 30 years of caring for older men, I have only cared for two men over the age of 80 who died from prostate cancer. I am quite sure that they both developed the cancer prior to turning 70. This man was diagnosed with prostate cancer after he turned 80. We stopped his antihormonal therapy and put him on testosterone, which we were ultimately able to stop when his body began producing its own. He regained his strength, and in the past 9 years, his PSA never went above 17! He recently celebrated his 97th birthday.

2.4 Geriatrics and the Individual

The geriatric approach to care is first and foremost based on the individual patient and their needs. We also have an obligation to look for evidence of the efficacy of our approach to patients. There is a growing body of literature regarding how care that we would deliver to a younger individual does not have the same outcomes in older adults. Until this changes, we have both a responsibility and an opportunity to look closely at our approach to the care of older individuals and respond accordingly.

With this in mind, in 1995 a group of geriatricians who worked in GeriMed of America's MedWise™ Centers came together to develop what essentially was a mission statement for how we approached the care of our patients. This became the MedWise™ Philosophy of Care. To this day, I believe it provides an excellent foundation for how clinicians should approach the care of older adults.

2.4.1   The MedWise™ Philosophy of Care

1. Focus on function (standard geriatric medical doctrine).
2. Focus on managing chronic disease(s) and developing chronic care treatment models. (As many older patients have one or more chronic illnesses, the management of chronic disease, versus the cure of such, is of paramount concern.)
3. Identify and manage psychological and social aspects of care. (It is quite often that psychosocial issues either directly or indirectly impact the health and well-being of a senior. The deterioration of a patient's social structure can lead to a hospitalization or decline in function. The awareness and management of these issues is a critical component of good geriatric care.)
4. Respect patient's dignity and autonomy. (A recognition of the paternalism that is still pervasive in medicine. We need to listen to our patients wishes and recognize the impact of illness and disability on a person's dignity.)
5. Respect cultural and spiritual beliefs (an oft forgotten aspect of the interpersonal relationship necessary for effective communication).
6. Be sensitive to the patients financial condition. (A patient's financial problems might lead to a lack of resources for effective care or an inability to buy medications or other supplies.)
7. Promote wellness. (Health promotion may have more importance in the ongoing physical well-being of the older individual. There is more and more literature demonstrating the benefits of exercise and good nutrition in the older patient.)
8. Listen and communicate effectively. (Too often it is the clinician doing most of the talking. We will only learn about our patients by listening to them.)
9. Patient-centered approach to care and customer-focused approach to service. (This was the most contentious discussion among our physicians but may be one of the most profound and important conclusions reached. The physician focuses on the patient in the exam room, but the office must treat the patient as a customer. Many seniors do not ask for help and will allow themselves to be pushed around in many healthcare systems. This can lead to delays in evaluation and treatment.)
10. Realistically promote optimism and hope. (This follows in the realm of respecting patient's dignity. We must be realistic with our patients, so as to guide them through the decision-making process.)
11. Team approach to care. (The hallmark of geriatric medical care is a team approach, recognizing the value of all members of the team in caring for the older patient.)

At GeriMed of America, our focus was on delivering the geriatric approach to care. It was, and will continue to be, necessary to develop a model of care around which to provide this approach. The model that we developed at GeriMed is essentially the same model that we used successfully at Senior Care of Colorado. The main tenets of this model are as follows.

2.4.2 Geriatric Medical Model of Care

1. Spend time with the patient. (This may be the hallmark of all that is geriatric medicine. Spending time with one's patient allows for the true development of a doctor/patient relationship that can be a partnership. The patient can trust and respect their primary care physician, and this trust is critical in the decision-making process that separates geriatricians from other physicians. Included in spending time with the patient is listening to all of the patient's complaints and not leaving them with a feeling that their questions have gone unanswered.)
2. High touch, low tech. (This is fairly obvious, but anecdotally, lots of tests and treatments are often counterproductive in the older patient. In this vein, doing less is often better and reduces iatrogenic complications.)
3. Focus on function and quality of life. (Fairly standard geriatric medical doctrine makes function and quality of life issues a focal point, rather than diagnosis, treatment, and cure. It also helps to focus the care plan and its evaluation in a way that is conducive to the patient's own understanding of complex issues.)
4. Practice the MedWise™ Philosophy of Care.

The final element that is necessary for the actual implementation of the geriatric approach to care is how to integrate the philosophy and the model of care into the actual practice. The following is a concise, albeit not completely comprehensive, summary of the key elements that we implemented into practice at GeriMed and subsequently with Senior Care of Colorado. I have always been a believer in the importance of integrating the approach to care into the workflow of the practice. The following principles are at the heart of this conceptual framework.

2.4.3 Geriatric Medical Approach to Practice

1. Aggressively avoid acute hospitalization in order to avoid iatrogenesis. (There is plenty of literature and experience demonstrating the risks of acute hospitalization. Many of the treatments that occur in the acute hospital, and even the intensive care unit, have no validated literature. The experience of many geriatricians would support the concept of conservative instead of aggressive treatment in the inpatient setting. While there are clear exceptions to this, many circumstances have no clear reason for aggressive management.)
2. Aggressively use office, home, attendant care, SNF, and other subacute levels of care as appropriate to improve patients quality of life and response to treatment. (Patients will do better in the most appropriate setting, with the home being the ideal setting if possible.)

3. Work to improve quality of care in skilled nursing facilities and home care by taking on active leadership roles in the delivery of care in those settings. (This is something that both GeriMed and Senior Care of Colorado did. By taking leadership roles throughout the entire continuum of care, we are better able to assure the highest quality of care for our patients.)

4. Use specialists appropriately; avoid fragmented care caused by multiple specialists. (Once again, there is very little literature supporting the benefit of specialists in a wide variety of disease states. Furthermore, there is a paucity of geriatric medical training in many of the subspecialties at this time. Some of GeriMed's own experiences in taking on large numbers of seniors would support the potential negative impact of unbridled specialty care on the older patient.)

5. Avoid polypharmacy. (Once again, the literature is very clear on this issue.)

6. Address advance directives in advance. (The literature has generally not supported the ability of physicians to effectively discuss advance directives with their patients. Our experience has proven otherwise. Given the time to talk to patients, and understanding the art of such discussions, they are often quite receptive to discussing these issues.)

7. Be firm, but fair, with "please doctor" requests. Don't change one's approach if it's not good for the patient. Keep the focus on delivering the most appropriate care. (Perhaps one of the most problematic areas for many of our physicians. Patients had gotten used to the way medicine has been practiced in the fee-for-service Medicare world. They are often used to seeing multiple specialists. When they are told that this might not be in their best interest, some patients resist. The important issue here is whether or not we believe in our model of care. If we do and this model discourages the fragmentation of care caused by patients seeing multiple specialists who may be lacking in geriatric medical training, then we must hold steadfastly to these principles. The vast majority of patients understand this, and the small minority that don't probably should not be seeing a geriatrician.)

This is the starting point of our journey into how to develop an effective business in the geriatric space. The rest of this book will be of no value if one doesn't agree with the principles laid out in this chapter. *You have to believe in the geriatric approach to care if you want to develop an effective geriatric business model!*

Matching Clinical Strengths to Revenue

3

The key to any successful business is to provide a quality product with excellent service. Geriatric practices are not only no exception to this important concept but should in fact be the rule. Clinicians must not only be encouraged to provide the best possible care but need to know up front that providing high-quality care is their primary goal. The service element is also critical for many reasons and becomes especially important with any increase in frailty and functional disabilities. We will discuss this much more in another chapter. Still, the major concern for clinicians trying to deliver geriatric care is how they will get paid. If I had a nickel for every time a doctor has told me that caring for Medicare beneficiaries was impossible because of inadequate reimbursement, I could retire again. Yet, this has been a consistent refrain from primary care physicians for many years and is clearly the crux of the issue of how to successfully provide geriatric medical care in the healthcare marketplace.

3.1 Evaluating Provider Reimbursement

Part of the challenge in evaluating provider reimbursement is that it has seemed to be a moving target. As an example, the infamous "SGR" provided an annual threat of significant cuts. This was finally "fixed" in early 2015. This methodology has been replaced by the future certainty of additional changes in the form of bundling and value-based reimbursement. At the same time, it is highly unlikely that basic fee-for-service reimbursement will completely disappear. This will become an important part of the discussion, as it is imperative to develop reimbursement strategies that span the gamut of possibilities. I believe that historically one of the reasons that geriatric practices have struggled is an overreliance on single-payment methodologies. This approach generally fails to take into account that the healthcare market as a whole exists in a world with multiple payment approaches. An overreliance on one method ignores the impact that other methods continue to have on the various players that a geriatrics practice encounters on a daily basis.

© Springer International Publishing Switzerland 2016   11
M. Wasserman, *The Business of Geriatrics*, DOI 10.1007/978-3-319-28546-7_3

While it may sound trite, if you don't believe that something is possible, then it probably won't happen. Starting with the belief that it is impossible to be financially viable in geriatrics will certainly prevent one from becoming successful. On the other hand, if one believes that it is possible, then the challenge is determining how to make it so. This is where most clinicians fail. Lacking a background in business, it can be difficult to figure out how to make a geriatrics practice profitable. Similarly, traditional business people who don't have a good understanding of geriatrics are also often unable to properly connect the dots in ways that bring profitability to a geriatrics practice. *Thus, the key to a financially viable geriatrics practice is melding an understanding of geriatrics and the continuum of care with sound business principles.*

3.2   Staying True to the Geriatric Approach to Care

The single most important underlying factor in the success of a geriatrics practice is that it stays true to the geriatric approach to care. Older adults appreciate a healthcare provider that cares about them. I have long wondered if this would be a generational issue, insofar as those that grew up during the depression tend to have a natural respect for doctors. There has been some concern that the baby boomers might be different, but from an observational perspective, I have come to see from my patients that as we age there is an almost natural evolution in our attitudes toward the aging process. While this book is not meant to be a treatise on the sociology of the aging process, there are certain observations that one makes over 30 years in the field. The older population may be singularly unique in their acceptance of physicians who demonstrate true concern about their quality of life and function.

Classic internal medicine training focuses on making a diagnosis and coming up with a treatment plan. The goal is often curative in nature, even when a cure is actually impossible. Geriatricians focus on maximizing function and quality of life. Multiple chronic diseases must be managed in a way that is most satisfying to the patient. The dichotomy of these two approaches cannot be overstated. When I first started practicing, I spent months trying to identify the source of a pain in one of my older patients. Visit after visit was unsuccessful in either delineating the cause or completely treating the symptoms. One day he said to me, "Doc, if we can't figure this out, let's go onto something else. I can live with this." While I would actually never stop trying to help him with this problem, this was a very informative experience. Older people are certainly adept at learning to live with a multitude of chronic illnesses. It is our job to make that process a little easier.

3.3   Palliative Care

The evolution of the field of palliative care should come as no surprise to anyone paying attention to today's healthcare marketplace. For a number of reasons, an approach that is second nature to most geriatricians has managed to become its own specialty. Unburdened from the baggage of ageism and negative perceptions of aging and geriatrics, the field of palliative care has found itself in the right place at the right time. Grant money and demonstration projects have allowed the field to show that this approach can be cost-effective while delivering satisfied patients. However, the field is now being challenged by the same issues that geriatricians have faced for years. How do palliative care providers get paid in a predominantly fee-for-service, procedurally based healthcare marketplace? The answers to that question should actually run parallel to the discussions covered in this book. At the same time, from both a marketing perspective and operationally, a geriatric practice must know how to demonstrate that the palliative care approach is an important aspect of the geriatric model of care.

3.4 The Importance of the Customer

While the geriatric approach to care is a key theme throughout this book, how to integrate that approach into a business is critical. One of the most contentious discussions during the development of GeriMed's Philosophy of Care™ was regarding whether to treat patients as customers. *The agreed upon compromise was that geriatrics focused on a patient-centered approach to care with a customer approach to service.* This solution is not to be taken lightly. In the exam room, the doctor-patient relationship is everything. This needs to be encouraged and highlighted, for both the benefit of the physician and the patient. Once the patient leaves the room, a focus on customer service must necessarily take over. There are many examples of how this takes hold. Arranging for home health follow-up can be critical in a patient who has been falling. Coordinating multiple tests and consults might also be challenging if a patient suffers from cognitive dysfunction. Another great example of the service component is how we deal with prior authorizations in today's increasing managed care environment.

When a physician is seeing a patient in the exam room and, based on their clinical experience and acumen, determines that a test or treatment is necessary, it should happen. I preface this with the caveat that I am speaking from the vantage point of a geriatrician who tends to be very holistic. *Once I have made my determination, it needs to be carried out. The patient should not be told that their workup or treatment can only occur if the insurance company approves it.* It might be necessary to explain that there are processes that need to take place to get approval, but it is incumbent upon the clinician and practice to do everything in their power to assure that their clinical judgment is carried out. I have heard far too many doctors complain about insurance company policies and being unable to get their patients the care that they need. On one hand, some of these might actually reflect the fact that many of these physicians were trying to order unnecessary tests. On the other hand, it may also have reflected a lack of willingness to fight for what they believe to be right.

This issue is very pertinent in today's healthcare world and might actually be the most contentious discussion in this book. There are certainly some interesting ironies. As I noted, I tend to be quite holistic. If I have a patient with a fever, cough, and egophony on lung exam, I might not even order a chest X-ray. If a patient has a classic progressive history of symptoms consistent with Alzheimer's disease over the course of a couple of years, there is no reason for a CT scan or an MRI. On the other hand, if I'm seeing an elderly patient who fell yesterday, hit their head, and is now displaying a sudden change in their neurological status, they need an urgent CT scan to rule out a subdural hematoma. Under such circumstances, we do not have time to get a prior authorization. It is a sad state of affairs that we have reached a point where we need to go through someone who doesn't even know our patient in order to get something done. However, the wanton abuse and misuse of tests and procedures has put us in this position. With that said, we must hold steadfast if we believe that our patient needs an urgent test or treatment.

3.5   Don't Take No for an Answer

It has been my experience that if I take the time to speak with an insurance company medical director and explain the clinical picture, there are usually no problems. On the rare occasion that I might run into a problem, I will ask the medical director if he or she is willing or able to take over the liability and care of my patient. The answer to that question is always no. It should not be surprising to find that many of these systems have been set up knowing that the primary care physician's office will not question a denial. It is not a surprising theme in this book that if the provider believes they can't do something, then they won't. While there are certain to be anecdotal experiences where the approach that I advocate for doesn't work, in my experience that has been extremely rare. *Administratively, the denials and the processes themselves create the cost savings that the insurance company is looking for.* Ironically, those cost savings are typically up front and short term and do not reflect a longer-term view of our patient's health care. That story is for another chapter or perhaps another book.

The existing methodology for reimbursing primary care physicians runs through the CPT coding system. This system was developed by the American Medical Association in the 1960s and expanded upon in the 1980s. Geriatric medicine board certification didn't even exist until 1988 and, even today, is limited to approximately 1 % of all physicians. It is not difficult to ascertain that a coding system that stops counting when one reaches four problems might not be adequate for geriatricians. With that said, the CPT codes have developed sets of rules that providers must abide by in order to code at various levels. This book is not meant to be an instructional treatise for coding, but the important take-home message is that one must know the rules in order to play by them.

3.6   Understand Coding

When we founded Senior Care of Colorado in 2001, it became readily apparent that we needed to understand the CPT coding system in order to get paid fairly for the care our clinicians provided to their patients. *Everyone at the time told us that this was impossible, but we did not accept that premise.* What we did shaped the future success of our practice. We studied the coding rules and we looked at how we delivered care to older adults. We then found ways to connect the two. While it seems relatively straightforward and simple, we believed then, and I believe now, that if necessary services cannot be provided for a fair price, then that system must ultimately fail. The knowledge that Medicare is a program that politicians will never allow to fail has always provided the impetus for seeking out effective ways to connect the dots between the approach to care and adequate reimbursement. For those who consider this either naive or wrong, I can only point to successful results as a response. Being very pragmatic, giving up is impractical, and giving in is just wrong from the perspective of professionalism.

With the advent of alternative payment methodologies, there will now be new opportunities to address the reimbursement issue. While we will discuss that shortly, it is important to reiterate that it is highly unlikely that fee-for-service payment will completely disappear in the near future. Furthermore, even those organizations and systems that receive bundled or capitated payments will probably continue to use fee-for-service methods for determining provider productivity and payment. In many ways, the complexity of the payment system is about to increase. This doesn't have to lead to problems, it just points to the need for comprehensive and thoughtful solutions.

Our ultimate solution to the CPT conundrum was to recognize the importance of time-based coding. The CPT codes allow for a clinician to bill in the office for face-to-face time spent with the patient, so long as more than 50 % of that time was spent in education and counseling. The reality of geriatrics is that if one spends a lot of time with a patient, by definition that visit will be dominated by education and counseling. I have bounced this concept off many of my colleagues over the past 20 years and rarely get a negative response. In the nursing home, the issue is a little different, but it still works. If more than 50 % of one's time is spent in coordinating care, then a visit can be billed based on time. Considering the fact that many nursing home residents have cognitive impairment, the time that one spends talking to the nurse and other staff will generally predominate the visit. Again, this book is not meant to be a coding treatise, but the point is that we realized that geriatricians will often see the need to spend time with patients, and we looked for a way to allow our providers to spend that time and be reimbursed for it. Alternative payment models will do well to recognize the importance of having clinicians spend time with patients and their families as they develop internal productivity metrics.

3.7 The Future Is Now

Are the new alternative payment models good for geriatrics? Absolutely! *In fact, these new methods provide a distinct path for the geriatric approach to care to explode in the coming years.* From personal experience in the 1990s with GeriMed of America and then with Senior Care of Colorado, there is no question that the geriatric approach is a very cost-effective one. The chapter on my experience in

Orlando, Florida, provides an instructive discussion of the development of a full risk model based on the geriatric approach to care coupled with a care coordination model. Ironically, while Senior Care of Colorado never took such risk, we certainly helped the local Medicare Advantage program reap profits through their relationship with our clinicians who followed a geriatric approach to care.

This is the future of healthcare. Those who pay attention to the geriatric approach to care will be well placed to succeed financially. Why has this not happened to a significant degree yet? Therein lies the rub. In fact, the HMOs of the 1990s and the subsequent Medicare Advantage plans have certainly had similar opportunities for financial success. Yet these successes have only occurred on a very limited basis. At the core of this issue is a costly approach to care that is very well ingrained in today's healthcare system.

It is ironic that as a geriatrician I have often been asked for evidence that the high-touch, low-tech approach to care that I espouse actually works. The irony is that much of the healthcare that is delivered today has not been scrutinized to the same degree. That is finally changing. The recent focus on value and quality is changing the conversation and appears to be altering the dynamics that have historically held the development of geriatrics in check. With that said, complacency in this area needs to be avoided. Just because we are headed in the right direction doesn't mean that there will not be many bumps on the road. The next chapter tells a story of how a geriatric approach to care can be successfully integrated into a full-risk practice model.

Taking Full Risk

4

It is a continuing theme of this book that we learn from our experiences. In the past 20 years, geriatricians have not had many opportunities to take significant financial risk based on their practice model. With the advent of a new focus on alternative payment models, these types of opportunities are about to increase dramatically. I have been fortunate to have had significant experience in this realm and will share the experience that shaped my knowledge and understanding of taking full financial risk with a large number of Medicare beneficiaries.

4.1 An Opportunity Arises

My immersion into practice management in the full-risk managed care setting started in May 1998. While attending the American Geriatrics Society's annual meeting, I ran into a colleague who told me that his nursing home company had some clinics in Orlando that they were looking to sell. Would GeriMed be interested? That question led to a follow-up phone call with the president of the operation that the nursing home company had set up in attempting to own and operate its own clinics. It turned out that they had acquired these clinics a couple of years earlier (their third owner over a short period of time) and had been losing a significant amount of money on their operations. These clinics had a past relationship with Humana and still cared for 3000 Humana Gold Medicare risk patients.

Three thousand Medicare risk patients translated roughly to 14 million dollars in potential revenue. The AAPCC (average adjusted per capita cost) in Orlando was about $500 per member per month, and with a 5 % reduction by HCFA and approximately 20 % off the top for the HMO, we would be left with almost 14 million dollars per year in which to care for our patients. This was the opportunity that GeriMed of America, Inc. had been looking for.

© Springer International Publishing Switzerland 2016
M. Wasserman, *The Business of Geriatrics*, DOI 10.1007/978-3-319-28546-7_4

4.2   Due Diligence

Dr. Jim Riopelle, our CEO, and Dennis Kuper, our CFO, took a trip down to Orlando in June to kick the tires and do GeriMed's form of "due diligence." What they found were four primary care offices that represented traditional doctor's practices. This meant physicians trying to see as many patients as possible in a day, referring patients out to specialists on a regular basis, and hospital utilization that was the norm in the Orlando market. Jim and I met with the physicians, and they seemed open to our approach to care. We identified two physicians in the group who essentially were the leaders.

The nursing home company wanted to "sell" us the practice and we wanted to "buy." Now it was just a matter of getting the deal done. Negotiations commenced and initially were to have been completed by July 1st. Final terms were not forthcoming and the negotiations dragged into August. GeriMed had its annual medical director's meeting in Keystone, Colorado. The two physicians from the existing practice were both invited and attended the meeting, even though the final negotiations had not been completed. We felt that it was essential to have them meet and interact with our other physicians to facilitate the transition process that was going to occur in Orlando. We had just begun working on our Clinical Glidepaths™, and this was a good opportunity to inculcate our ideas into the new group. This is an important concept when it comes to physician engagement. Physicians need the shelter and comfort of other physicians. Introducing these doctors to other physicians who practiced with GeriMed was a key element in bringing them on board.

There were a few different "deals" that had to get completed simultaneously in order to make the whole deal work. First, the 3000 Humana patients were essentially worthless unless they fell under a full-risk contract. This meant completing a contract with Humana for a full-risk arrangement. This wasn't that difficult insofar as Humana wanted to assure the continuity of care for patients who participated in their plan. However, they had a few requirements that we had to think hard about. One of these was the use of a hospitalist group that they had an ownership stake in. It is notable that the hospitalist industry was just starting to ramp up at this time. The hospitalist company had been organized by an internist in Texas, whose concept was that by focusing the acute hospital care on a small group of providers, one could achieve improved utilization. They had been successful in Texas and some other markets and had been trying to develop their operations in Orlando. We had a couple of concerns about using this group. One, they were not geriatricians and therefore would probably not understand our approach to care. Two, they cost too much.

We also had to make a decision on how we wanted to manage claims and utilization management. There was a relatively new Medical Service Organization (MSO) in the Orlando market. They were trying to organize physicians in the market in order to gain more clout with Humana and other HMOs. It sounded like a good idea, but was going to cost us 6 % of our revenue. While at our medical director's meeting, I spent most of the time on the telephone dealing with the final stages of our negotiations with the nursing home company and the MSO. I kept trying to figure out what we were going to get for our 6 % and ultimately convinced them to lower the number to 4 ½%. Still, it didn't feel right.

Finally, there was Humana. Being one of the largest HMOs in the country, they represented a formidable presence. They wanted an exclusive relationship with us. While this opportunity was the best one we had as an organization to date, tying ourselves to one HMO would have been like tying our hands and feet behind our back. This was not an area for compromise.

We closed the deal on August 15, 1998, retroactive to August 1st. We essentially had already owned the operations for 3 weeks by the time we first went down to Orlando the following week. The goal of that trip was to meet with the staff of each office, meet with the physicians, meet with the people from the nursing home company to close out a few details, meet with the MSO, and meet with Humana.

4.3   Decisions to Make

Running a primary care doctor's office is perhaps one of the most difficult tasks which exist in the world of business. Many patients leave a physician's practice, not because of the doctor, but because of their staff. I have often wondered if there is a genetic trait that leads office staff to protect their physicians. On the other hand, it may be that physicians, knowingly or unknowingly, present an aura which leads staff to try to protect them. Whatever the etiology, this behavior often leads to delays in setting up appointments and responses to phone calls. When running a medical office, this is a key management element to be aware of. Training the staff to place the focus on the patient as a customer is a high priority. It is also a priority that requires constant vigilance.

Next was the issue of cost and budget. GeriMed had always professed to have an expensive primary care approach. This does not mean that we had the ability or desire to waste money. We especially didn't want to waste money and resources in the wrong place. The place to spend money was where it related to direct patient care in order to have the greatest impact on the quality and cost-effectiveness of that care.

The nursing home company had in place a whole corporate infrastructure, which included an entire executive layer, which clearly was not going to be needed. There was then another layer of "middle management" and finally three office managers for the four clinics. We had discussions with the regional administrator and ultimately decided to offer her a position. Fortunately, she declined, and we were forced to get organized without a person in this capacity. This would mean that administrative oversight and responsibility would fall directly upon our Vice President of Operations. His background was in accounting and the seafood business, although in the past few years, he had become very knowledgeable about the hospital-based cost reimbursement model. Managed Medicare as we were about to dive into the waters was relatively new to him. On the other hand, I had thought myself knowledgeable about managed care, with a background of 5 years at Kaiser Permanente in Southern California. I was only beginning to learn how little I knew.

We went down to Orlando with Ray Delisle, our Chief Operating Officer. I have always said that Ray has more business experience in his little finger than I will ever have. Ray masterfully led our meetings at each clinic, explaining how we were going to have to earn their trust. This is an important concept when taking over an existing practice. You can't bulldoze over people, even if you are now their employer. You have a responsibility to demonstrate through your actions that they should put their trust in you. Keep in mind, these clinics had been through three owners in the immediate past. To them, why would we be any different? We explained our model to the office staff, but realized that only time was going to allow for us to instill GeriMed's model into practice.

4.4   Meeting the Physicians

We met with the physicians. If we were going to be successful, we were going to have to affect the way these physicians practiced. They were all internists, but there were no true geriatricians in the group. I explained the geriatric medical model, but could tell that they didn't quite understand it. As our model was partially based upon a team approach to care which includes care coordination, we had a decision to make. Do we hire care coordinators? What should their background be? How many do we hire? Keeping in mind that the operation was losing a lot of money when we took it on, this decision had financial implications all the way around. When it came down to it, the question needed to be posed, what was our model and did we believe in it?

In the years since my experience in Orlando, I have had many opportunities to make decisions that required a judgment about taking the best approach to improving the quality of care that we deliver to patients. I have also interacted with many other healthcare businesses that have had to make similar decisions. *This is ultimately the major tipping point for developing a successful business model for delivering geriatric care. You've got to believe in the geriatric approach to care and an integrated care coordination model.* Generally, others will neither understand nor appreciate either of these. There will be resistance and responding to any push back is key to the success of the practice. This is true not only of physicians, but of everyone who works in the practice.

One of the first things that we began to do upon our arrival was to meet with our physicians every week and begin the educational process of what geriatric medicine was all about and what our approach to care was. To this end, we went about developing a one-page summary sheet that pulled together some very basic facts about our model and our approach to care. These were covered in Chap. 2.

4.5   Focus on the Geriatric Model of Care

In our weekly physician meetings, we pounded on the basics of our model on a regular basis. One of the tools we used was to identify sample cases and use them to describe and highlight the geriatric medical model. Our next step was to hire a geriatrician who could act in the capacity of a peer to influence and educate the other physicians in the group. Fortunately, the name of the only fellowship-trained geriatrician practicing in Orlando was brought to my attention by one of the physicians in the practice. I quickly set up an interview with this geriatrician. It was obvious immediately that we were of the same ilk as geriatricians and understood and believed in the geriatric model of care. Interestingly, at this time I had no idea how we would structure the pay of our physicians, and he came on board on a handshake based on our general understanding of the model and trust in each other as fellow geriatricians. He was to prove instrumental in supporting the educational process and acting to affect his peers in the group. We soon realized that we would be undergoing some further attrition and began to seek out another geriatrician. Dr. Clemencia Rasquinha would join us in December. She was a fellowship-trained geriatrician who I had hired to work in one of GeriMed's hospital-based MedWise™ Centers in New Jersey. Ironically, the hospital did not appreciate what they had, and their loss proved to be our gain.

4.6   Give and Take

While most of our physicians didn't want to use a hospitalist group, this was not going to be a decision that we could make easily or lightly. Humana was quite insistent on our using the hospitalist company, and their having a stake in the company certainly influenced that stance. From the beginning, our concern was that this hospitalist company was made up of internists and not geriatricians. Furthermore, they were definitely expensive. They were charging a capitated rate and then would get capitated bonus dollars based on utilization improvement. Unfortunately, the "improvement" was already at the utilization rate that our group was running at. I had also had some history at Kaiser with the hospitalist concept and had been less than impressed with the methodology at that point in time. The positives were geographic coverage and a smaller group of physicians to manage. The negatives were physicians whose primary focus was the hospital (understanding the possibilities of care throughout the continuum might be lacking), lack of direct oversight, and the addition of yet another corporate/administrative layer.

The bottom line was that Humana wanted us to use the hospitalists and we wanted a nonexclusive relationship in the market. This would probably be the major compromise in our negotiations. The coming year would add many new insights and experiences to this decision process, and a year later we would once again be discussing the same issue with Humana.

It was clear from the beginning of our arrival in Orlando that there were significant issues with the practice in regard to specialty utilization. Jim Riopelle's initial chart review had identified specialty referral patterns as an issue which we needed to get our arms around quickly. There were also issues regarding existing capitated relationships with some specialty providers. The cardiologists were apparently unhappy with their capitated dollar amount, as were the surgeons. We quickly set up meetings with both groups and agreed to raise their capitation rates. We didn't try to negotiate. It was our intent to make sure that the specialists were happy with their capitation rate and at the same time educate our physicians about the proper utilization of specialists. It would make no sense to capitate specialists and then overutilize them, as this would lead to a spiraling effect of increased utilization of other services and ultimately a request by the specialists to further increase the capitation rate. On the other hand, under a capitated relationship, the specialists would be encouraged to appropriately utilize and care for our patients. While we would have occasional differences and disagreements with the cardiologists and surgeons over the year, the relationships actually worked quite well. We also had capitated relationships with two orthopedic surgeons, an oncology group (which was quite important) and a gastroenterology group. We would still have some issues with the oncologists as it related to our feeling of responsibility for managing our patients from a primary care standpoint, but this would be dealt with the same way we dealt with all problems which related to specialists.

4.7   Specialty Capitation

We continued to have discussions at a corporate level regarding the topic of subspecialty capitation. By capitating specialists, we were in essence limiting our upside potential of reducing specialty utilization. At the same time, we were limiting our downside potential of excessive specialty utilization. Furthermore, specialists will also drive other areas of utilization, including testing and hospitalizations. This is a notable concept. Traditionally, Medicare expenditures relating to hospital care run in the range of 35–40 % of overall spending. It is ultimately the ability to limit hospital utilization and the resulting costs that has the biggest impact on a full-risk endeavor. Having good relationships with particular specialty groups can be quite conducive to cooperation in educating specialists in the nuances of geriatric medicine. It was also consistent with GeriMed's philosophy of being a physician-friendly organization. Nevertheless, from a business standpoint, we would continue to evaluate the cost-benefit of specialty capitation.

The approach we would take each time a disagreement developed with a particular specialty group was to set up a meeting and discuss our relationship as soon as possible. We would typically begin these meetings with the reminder that they were the specialty group that we had chosen to work with, that we enjoyed working with them, and that occasionally problems might develop in any relationship. We reminded them of our desire to grow in the market and to ultimately bring them even more business with our growth.

4.8   Information System Decision

One of the first decisions we had to make was what to do from an information system perspective. The nursing home company had spent a million dollars in licensing an information system, which didn't sound to us like it delivered what we needed. I had been responsible for overseeing the development of GeriMed's Care Management System (CMS). This process had been very frustrating at the time, and

CMS 98, as it was called, was months late from being rolled out. Nevertheless, this was it! Either our system was going to work or it wasn't. We had learned the lesson of not setting expectations for an upgrade without expecting delays. The CMS had been maligned by many at the time for this reason, and in fact, there was dissension in our IS department. The acquisition would ultimately prove to have been a major turning point in the development of the CMS.

From a decision-making perspective, sometimes one just has to suck it up and make a decision. Some of my best mentors have reminded me that there is no such thing as a good or bad decision. You make your decision and deal with the consequences! We knew that we needed an information system. Our homegrown system was undergoing growing pains, but it was ours. Looking back, our decision doesn't seem too surprising. We decided that we were going to use our own information system and that CMS 5.0 (as it was now called) would be rolled out in Orlando. We knew that we were essentially piloting our new version, replete with bugs, in our most important project to date.

Yet, this was our system and either it was going to work or we needed to get another computer system. Surprisingly, the staff in the clinics took to the system very well. They had suggestions and complaints, but many of the staff stated that the system was better than any other they had previously used. We tracked the suggestions and ultimately folded them into our next upgrade. I found the ability to walk into an office and pull up random patients on the computer system to be an effective means of evaluating the care being delivered in the office. Furthermore, we were able to use the "Referral Face Sheet" as an effective means of evaluating specialty referrals. This information was then fed back during our physician meetings in the form of an educational process.

4.9 Care Coordination

I had been in Orlando for a few weeks when I realized that physician education alone, or Geriatric Utilization Management, would not address the broader issues. Did we believe in the interdisciplinary team approach that we had broached as a company? Did we believe in one care coordinator per 750–1000 seniors? If we didn't, what had we been doing with our lives? What was the purpose of our company? The decision was easy. We would invest $250,000 (annual salaries) on four care coordinators. The initial reaction from our management team was "how can we afford to spend this much money on an operation that is presently losing money?" Our final answer was, "how can we afford not to?" The ad was placed and I began interviewing people for the job. Fortunately, four people fell out of the sky. Two were nurses, one from the hospital and another from our Winter Park office. Two were social workers, one with a nursing home background and the other from a community social services background. I explained our model to them and everyone seemed to feel that this was a job made in heaven! I also pointed out that they were going to be part of a groundbreaking opportunity, proving the worth and the efficacy of the geriatric care coordination model! I will readily admit to challenging them that the success of our program, and their jobs, depended on their success. This is another key component in working toward the successful implementation of a geriatric model of care. *Fire up the troops and have them own the approach to care!*

The four care coordinators started about the same time. We set up a weekly meeting schedule to discuss cases and problems. We did not have any guidelines to go on, and I decided that it was time to develop some. It was at this time that I called the nurse who had taught me most of what I knew about care coordination. Her name was Shirley Alcalde, and she had been my care coordinator at the geriatric consultation clinic that I started at Kaiser. Her background had been as a UM nurse with Cigna in the early 1980s and then as a discharge planner with Kaiser. Previously, she had experience in the nursing home industry as a Director of Nursing and was quite knowledgeable about the continuum of care. I had originally considered hiring her in Denver as my care coordinator 4 years earlier, but had been talked out of it due to our belief at the time in a pure social work model of care coordination (our belief had obviously changed). I called Shirley, and we began working on developing guidelines to define the role of our care coordinators. These guidelines were then passed on to our care coordinators in Orlando. I believe that they read them and automatically understood them, because we had been fortunate in hiring people who had an intuitive understanding of our model and approach to care. It is doubtful that these guidelines were referred to on a regular basis, but that is probably not important. These guidelines are found in Chap. 18.

Both Jim Riopelle and I came from a utilization management background. Jim first encountered UM as a medical director in the early 1980s with Qual-Med, and I began getting involved in UM with Kaiser in the early 1990s. Jim's experience was that traditional UM did not work in the Medicare population. My experience was that there needed to be a geriatric medical bent to the process, but that proper systems in place are also needed which are readily accessible and utilized the entire continuum of care. In the early 1980s we were able to achieve acute "days/1,000" in the low 800s with Southern California Kaiser using a process described as "care coordination rounds." This process entailed a geriatrician rounding daily with a social worker, discharge planner, home health liaison, and the primary nurses. The geriatrician would interact directly with the PCP. Geriatric consultation would be performed on an ad hoc basis in the hospital. We certainly were missing the ability to impact patients prior to the hospital admission, and I always felt that given the proper approach, acute hospital days in the range of 500–600 could be achieved.

4.10 Hospital Days per Thousand

Prior to our acquiring the facilities, the previous owners had begun its own utilization management process. Years before, their days/1000 had run at a rate of 1280. Interestingly, this was average for the market. They had a utilization nurse who had been working with one of their physicians. By the time we went down toward the end of August, the month of August was already a lost month in terms of affecting utilization. The month of September involved numerous meetings, and we essentially kept the existing UM process going during that time. It wasn't until October that I began getting more involved in looking at acute hospital care and began the "battle" with the hospitalists in trying to educate them about acute inpatient geriatric medical care. We quickly identified a myriad number of issues with the hospitalists. These included the following:

1. Extensive use of specialists. (This is not an atypical problem for hospitalist groups, depending on how they are incentivized. When we entered into such relationships, we tried to align incentives so that they would have some risk for Part B costs as well.)
2. High use of tests. (Again, often seen as a way of getting people out of the hospital quickly, but not always necessary in the geriatric population. The adage of only doing a test if the result will guide therapy is a basic tenet of good geriatric care.)
3. Lack of aggressive monitoring of planned discharges.
4. Lack of weekend continuity of care. (This continued to be a problem for the entire period of our relationship.)
5. Poor communication with family for patients in the ICU, especially on weekends. (Many of the hospitalists were relatively new out of training and did not have the experience, nor the training in the art of these types of discussions.)
6. Nonaggressive approach to ER decisions to admit. (Hospitalists are typically more familiar with the acute hospital care setting and are not as knowledgeable or comfortable with the delivery of care in other settings.)
7. Poor communication with the primary care physicians.
8. Could be more aggressive with use of subacute care initially.
9. Need for additional training in discussing patient wishes.
10. Need to take more responsibility for interacting with and discussing plan of care with specialists.

We began to deal with these issues in November and by December instituted daily rounds in the hospital with chart review. Over the next 2 months, our care coordinator and I rounded on a regular basis. I continued to work closely with the hospitalists in attempting to educate them and point out alternatives for disposition and a geriatric medical approach to care. Of note, our hospital-based care coordinator had been trained in a more traditional utilization management nurse approach, and part of the process was to educate her about the differences in the geriatric medical utilization management approach.

For interest, I have included a sample summary from our heavy direct UM (with examples).

4.10.1 Hospital Rounds 12/7

A1. "Baseline condition" noted in chart, plan was to keep treating with intravenous antibiotics and watching in hospital. Spoke to patient and family to verify and spoke to hospitalist, will d/c today with home care and care coordinator follow-up (*2–3 days saved*).

This patient was very interesting, insofar as they had COPD, and while they "looked bad," they were in fact at their baseline condition. *This is a common problem when patients are being cared for by other physicians who do not know them.*

A2. Psych patient, needs transfer if CT negative, hospitalist hasn't seen yet— 12:45 pm, admit 12/5, not yet seen by psych. Psych called over the weekend, but due to miscommunications, didn't get seen, no medical issues, discharge dependent on psych, but no aggressive follow-up of this over the weekend (*1–2 days lost*).

A3. Followed by pulmonologist's NP, hospitalist seems to be following their plan, CT ordered, possible bronchoscopy, plan based on results of CT and bronchoscopy is not clear, patient also with a saphenous DVT. Spoke to patient and family at length. Patient wants to go home and is aware of risk/benefit. Care coordinator home visit follow-up arranged (*2–3 days saved*).

This case was remarkable in that it didn't take any prompting whatsoever to get the patient to tell us that she didn't even want to be in the hospital. *It is an important lesson in keeping patients out of the emergency room for any routine problem, because the ER visit can lead to an unnecessary admission.*

4.10.1.1 Hospital Rounds 12/8

B1. Urinary tract infection, Alzheimer's disease, falling at home, admitted to hospital. Brought into hospital directly. Our physician knew about the admission. Could have been admitted to SNF directly (*1 day lost—our responsibility*).

This was a valuable learning case for one of our own physicians, who was just learning the potential of using other settings of care. The good news was that this only happened one time, demonstrating the value of immediate education.

A2. Still in hospital CT negative, awaiting psych at noon.

B2. Cath and CABG, PCP not notified (*1 day lost*).

B3. MICU, ischemic bowel, sepsis, CRF, COPD, etc. Prognosis poor—no one talking to wife about issues. No clear discussion of patient's wishes and what's going on daily (*potential for lost days*).

This was proven to be an ongoing issue.

B4. 74 years old with h/o BPH, in for suprapubic prostatectomy.

B5. pod#4 for mass and SBO excision, clear liquid, and oral analgesics today. Talked to hospitalist, who will talk to surgeon about discharge today.

Additional note on SNF patient (not ours, but following in SNF): Pt at SNF, hospitalist admitted, sent back to SNF on Monday with intravenous hydration, patient severely demented, family confused about life support issues. Admitted to us in SNF. Issues regarding admitting demented pts with NG tubes and no clear family discussion regarding long-term issues.

4.10.1.2 Hospital Rounds 12/9

B5. Still in hospital, hospitalist "couldn't reach surgeon," d/c today (*1 day lost*).

C1. CP/syncope—EtOH 316, negative CK and troponin, binge drinker, negative persantine 4/97, h/o hiatal hernia and ulcers, smoker. CT scan and Doppler ordered for unclear reasons, ECG ok, patient to have stress test.

B3. Still sick. Our physician to see today—wife has stated to us that patient wouldn't want to be like this, but she may have trouble letting go (*days saved*).

C2. Infected wound—plan for discharge to SNF.

C3. In TCC, hospitalist notes do not comment on functional status—this is the key reason to see patient in TCC. Could review entire case–has anyone asked about pt's wishes? Had been getting Haldol. *I spoke to cousin in Connecticut about patient's wishes. Wife died several months ago and he had been unhappy since. Would definitely not want aggressive treatment if his future function and quality of life were considered to be poor. Cousin would like to see him moved closer to them for custodial comfort care (multiple SNF days lost, and a number of SNF days saved, possible lost days during hospital admission).*

C4. Previous CVA, decline recently after hospitalization on 11/20, SNF stay, d/c home on Saturday for presumed PT, didn't get seen for 3 days, seen 12/8 by PT, daughter felt something was wrong, care coordinator did home visit, weakness on left side that am, spoke to our physician, decision to direct admission—hospitalist not notified, had pre-cert, went to hospital that night due to change in status, Dx with CVA. Into hosp for 1 day and back to SNF. Family knows pt having multiple CVAs, will be custodial.

4.10.2 Hospital Rounds 12/10/1998

D1. 92-year-old female, fractured left wrist 1 week ago, ORIF today, day surgery, alert, lives in retirement community.

D2. Was in X-ray having a barium enema, nausea, and chest discomfort, admitted for chest pain, seen by hospitalist, can go home today.

C1. Stress test, heart cath, PTCA, stent placed. Needs F/U with our physicians.

B3. Hospice called in to see him today, pulled everything, no further dialysis, our physicians spoke to wife, considering pulling life support.

C2. Needs debridement.

C3. Working on getting to Connecticut; take off skilled.

4.10.2.1 Hospital Rounds 12/14
C3.Going wed on med-flight

Everyone else ok today

4.10.2.2 Hospital Rounds 12/15
E1. 88 years old s/p MI, CP, seen by cardiologist, hospitalist, comfort measures, still in hospital (*1 day lost*).

E2. COPD exacerbation.

E3. CP, I'm noting that everyone with chest pain sees a cardiologist—H&P reviewed, MI has been ruled out. Was admission appropriate? Spoke to cardiologist, who agrees that patient probably didn't need to be admitted (*1 day lost*).

E4. Unresponsive in bathroom at home, independent—nothing happened on Sunday. Doppler/CTs, Echo, EEG, neuro consult yesterday, set up for d/c today. New onset Sz, syncope, perhaps, looks fine—massive w/u and extra day in hosp. No need for neuro consult (*1 day lost, consult not necessary*).

E5. ECG changes, seen by hospitalist, previous w/u, med adjustment, out today. Not clear why not d/c yesterday (*1 day lost*).

E6. Should have been scoped over the weekend (*possible lost days*).

4.10.2.3 Hospital Rounds 12/16

F1. Acute renal failure on chronic, nephrology consult, most likely volume depletion.

F2. Prolapsed hemorrhoid.

4.10.2.4 Hospital Rounds 12/18

F1. Acute renal failure on chronic, nephrology consult, most likely volume depletion. "Watching numbers." Tried calling physician, out due to family emergency (*possible lost days*).

G2. OB pt – needed terbutaline pump—wasn't being case managed by Humana.

4.10.2.5 Hospital Rounds 12/21

H1. D/c order written yesterday! Was to be d/c after being seen by a cardiologist (note written underneath the cardiology note!). Pt not d/c! No apparent follow-up to assure that patient was discharged (*1 day lost*).

H2. Exp lap surgery.

H3. Gastrectomy.

4.10.2.6 Hospital Rounds 12/22

I1. Angina, seen by cardiologist yesterday, pt transferred from Florida east ER to Florida south! Were trying to keep in Florida system. Spoke to hospitalist who notes he has drifted to using cardiology for most patients with cardiac problems. Other physician said pt should have gone yesterday! (*1 day lost*).

I2. Fever, out of area/Dr. Our physician to speak to Dr. Spoke to hospitalist—son having trouble coping, daughter chose facility.

I3. Perforated bowel in Germany—we don't know anymore.

E6. Admit to SNF, h/o CVAs, working on NH issues/daughter has not called care coordinator back. Poor family support.

H2. pod #1, exp lap, removed mass.

4.10.2.7 Hospital Rounds 12/23

J1. Nosebleed and HTN.

I2. Out of area, ready to go—SNF has accepted. Care coordinator has put a lot of time into this case determining the patients' status and arranging for SNF placement. I called the physician, who was not planning on discharging the patient until Friday. He states that he will d/c tomorrow morning. Hospitalist involvement has been minimal as their medical director is out of town.

4.10.2.8 Hospital Rounds 12/28

K1. Sepsis, MICU, h/o non-small cell lung ca—consult for pulmonary, oncology, and ID, pulmonary planning to bronchoscopy tomorrow, PCP no longer with our group. I spoke with hospitalist regarding having him speak to family to delineate all of patient's wishes in preparation for patient's status going bad. Also, asked hospitalist to speak to pulmonologist to delineate the need for bronchoscopy—what is the intended outcome and what will be done with results, due to risk of patient requiring ventilator support after bronchoscopy and possibly never coming off vent (*potential for lost days*).

I2. D/c yesterday—2/27.

L1. Florida Hospital, pneumonia (admit 12/26), from ALF, on IV ABX, had been declining, sl temp today, hemodynamically stable? SNF? As both initial and present alternative. Temp on 102.7 on admission, but other vitals ok. Patient is DNR and guardian, who we spoke to, states he would not want very aggressive treatment. Patient will go to SNF today after our intervention (*1–2 days lost 1–2 days saved*).

This intensive period of geriatric medically focused UM appeared to have a positive effect. Our acute hospital utilization during this 2-month period of time dropped into the 500-day range (including the avoidable days!). This also coincided with our outpatient care coordination process and the hiring of two fellowship-trained geriatricians.

4.11 Negotiating with Hospitals

One of the other major challenges in healthcare is negotiating fair rates with hospitals and ancillary service providers. This area makes up an interesting chapter in our Orlando development. Unfortunately, a lot of the time and energy that we put into this arena was probably not constructive, although it could be argued that our interest in the area may have had some impact on the market as a whole.

When we arrived on the scene, our primary hospital was Lucerne Hospital, ironically (from GeriMed's past history), owned by Columbia. There were rumblings as to renegotiations between Humana and Columbia that might make their per diem rates less attractive. Also, our physicians had some questions as to Lucerne's ability to work in tandem with our approach to care. Some of our physicians suggested that we look at other possibilities in the market, and Princeton Hospital came up as one possibility. The Princeton Hospital was a hospital in Orlando that had been on the ropes for years. They were hungry and eager to work out a relationship. In fact, our business might keep them from having to close their doors. They were in a less than desirable location, and a number of our subspecialists did not go there. Nevertheless, they were offering excellent rates and a desire to work with us on developing an inpatient geriatric unit. Acute Care of the Elderly (ACE) units were only at the beginning of their development nationally, and we saw an opportunity to create one. The other hospitals in the area had no interest. Ironically, this is the one area that I have never been successful. The business case for an ACE unit is actually quite solid, but hospitals were and still are very difficult to convince. Anyway, by opening negotiations with another hospital, we had the opportunity to show the rest of the market that we were willing to bring our business elsewhere.

It is worth noting that when one is operating in a relatively small community (which Orlando was), whatever one says or does is known by most of that community within 24 h. Suffice it to say, within a day of our initial discussions with Princeton, others were aware. Without dragging this chapter out too long, nothing ultimately came of our negotiations with Princeton, and they folded almost a year later. In the meantime, our relationship with Lucerne actually improved significantly, and our ability to manage our hospital patients improved. The take-home message here is never say or do anything that you don't mind others knowing about. At the same time, be aware that having others know who you are talking to might influence their negotiating stance.

4.12   In the Middle of Giants

In January, it became clear that Humana and Columbia were at odds on their contract negotiations. Humana wanted us to shift our inpatient care to Florida Hospital. We resisted for a variety of reasons, the primary of which was our feeling that we would have less control over hospital utilization at Florida Hospital. On the other hand, we were not improving Humana's hand in decreasing business to Lucerne and improving their negotiating stance. We held out until the end of February. Humana and Columbia had until the end of March to come to an agreement, and we decided to throw our support behind Humana in March, shifting our admissions to Florida Hospital (we were right about the difficulty managing our patients there). Just prior to midnight on March 31, Humana and Columbia came to terms on a per diem contract. Unfortunately, just a few months later, Columbia sold Lucerne Hospital to Orlando Regional Health System. The saga of dealing with hospital contracts continued throughout our time in the market and is always the most challenging issue.

There are a few schools of thought on the importance of good hospital contracts. Traditional wisdom notes the high percentage of costs which relate to inpatient hospital care. This school of thought dictates the need for reasonable per diem contracts. There is a geriatric medical viewpoint which sees the acute hospital as a dying breed, with more care shifted to skilled nursing facilities, home care, and outpatient care. This school of thought focuses more on improving care in these other realms. It would be necessary to reduce hospital utilization below 500 days/1000 before we could afford to be less concerned about the costs of hospital care. Nevertheless, we thought that this was an obtainable goal.

GeriMed had always felt that it was critical to be able to manage patients throughout the entire continuum of care. Our model had always necessitated extensive involvement in skilled nursing facilities. We aggressively pursued nursing home medical directorships which allowed us to impact the quality of care in skilled nursing facilities to our satisfaction. Over the course of the first year of our operations in Orlando, we had mixed success in achieving these goals. However, as our at-risk population grew, the interest from the nursing facilities had increased. The "old days" of nursing facilities looking for physicians just to provide medical services for custodial long-term care patients were going fast. These physicians did not provide for a new population of patients, nor did they address the rapidly expanding arena of skilled/subacute care. With the advent of the PPS (Prospective Payment System), there was a critical need for physician-led support and insight into the management of high-acuity skilled patients. Furthermore, the daily per diem rates paid for managed care patients had suddenly become more attractive to the nursing home industry.

We insisted from the beginning that we continue to care for our patients admitted to skilled nursing facilities, and this worked well for us. We worked out an arrangement with the hospitalist company which allowed us to perform our own subacute care. As I note in another chapter, hospitalists generally don't function well in the nursing facility environment.

Any discussion of utilization issues must include home care, home infusion, and DME. Most HMOs have historically not addressed these arenas adequately. Our model depends on the ability to shift care to the most appropriate setting, and these ancillary services provide critical support for our model. This is why we were concerned when Humana told us that they had developed a capitated arrangement with another company. This other company would provide a "middle-man" function for the aforementioned services.

4.13   Aligning Incentives

Aligning incentives was a hallmark of GeriMed's contracting philosophy. In this case, we were worried that a capitated provider of ancillary services would be incentivized to withhold services. On the other hand, we knew that only physicians could order these services and that a physician's order could not be countermanded by a nonphysician, or so we thought. When our care coordinators started telling us that services that we thought were necessary were being denied or not provided in a timely fashion, we immediately brought the issue to the attention of Humana's medical director. We effectively applied the very important practice of documenting all of these instances, and Humana was very cooperative in dealing with these problems over the course of time. We ultimately achieved a fairly decent operational relationship with the ancillary provider.

It was notable that in the first couple of months of operations, our acute hospital utilization was approximately 1000 days/1000, and by the end of the first year, we had reduced that to approximately 600–700 days/1000. As to be expected in a geriatric practice, our skilled nursing utilization went from approximately 500 days/1000 to about 600–700 days/1000. Nevertheless, our blended utilization was still running about 30–40 % less than when we had acquired the practice.

After 1 year in the Orlando market, we had achieved solid utilization and financial results indicating the success of our model. Humana was satisfied to the extent of bringing us to the attention of other Humana regions which led to new business. In fact, it wasn't long before our four clinics in Orlando grew to a total of ten clinics between Tampa and Daytona.

One of the fascinating aspects of looking back at the success that we had in Central Florida was that it predated "risk-adjusted" payment methodologies. Being a practice that focused solely on Medicare beneficiaries, we were always prone to negative selection bias. Frail older patients would tend to gravitate to a primary care geriatric practice. The fact that we were financially successful despite having a negative selection bias was and still is a profound statement as to the viability of a geriatric practice model.

The Psychology of Geriatricians

5

I have often likened managing a group of physicians to herding gnats. The reason is simple. People are all different. The uniqueness of an individual's DNA assures us that any two people will be different. The ultimate impact of these differences is that each person reacts to stimuli in their own unique way. On the other hand, there are also a number of common traits that people share. Are they introverted or extroverted? Are they passive or aggressive? Are they rigid or flexible? Identifying these similarities and differences is an important factor in the hiring and management of clinicians.

Over many years I have had the opportunity to interact with many physicians, nurse practitioners, and physician assistants. I have hired them, fired them, and dealt with their personal problems and work habits. I have known physicians trained from an allopathic perspective as well as osteopaths. I've worked with physicians with a background in family medicine and internal medicine. I've known geriatricians who were board certified and those who weren't. Before discussing the psychology of geriatricians, however, I'm going to start this chapter by contrasting geriatricians with another group of physicians that I have encountered over the last 25 years. They form an excellent point of comparison. These are physicians who have chosen the field of hospital medicine.

5.1 The Hospitalist Comparison

Over the past 25 years, a new specialty was formed, and with it, a new group of physicians known as hospitalists has evolved. When I first started practicing, it was commonplace for a physician to see their own patients in the hospital every day. Today, this traditional approach has been replaced by one that seemingly makes sense from an efficiency perspective. We now have physicians who spend all of their time working in acute hospitals. One might imagine this to be a fairly high-stress

© Springer International Publishing Switzerland 2016   33
M. Wasserman, *The Business of Geriatrics*, DOI 10.1007/978-3-319-28546-7_5

position. Similarly, it would seem to be associated with a clinician who likes making immediate diagnoses and decisions. How do hospitalists deal with the more gradual approach that is necessary in caring for those with multiple chronic diseases?

Frail older adults often require observation, rather than immediate action. They need a clinician who will pay attention to factors such as their socioeconomic status. There also tends to be a lack of evidence-based knowledge available to guide the treatment of the frail elderly. Geriatrics leans far more to the art of medicine rather than the science. A high-touch, low-tech approach to care defines the way a geriatrician works. This is a very different approach than many physicians take in today's healthcare environment. One of the reasons that I have chosen to compare geriatricians with hospitalists is to illustrate the differences in how they would approach a patient.

I mentioned earlier in this book how I first experienced the hospitalist concept while with Kaiser in the early 1990s. My next experience was described in the preceding chapter about our experience developing a geriatrics practice in Orlando. It was obvious early on in both of those settings that the approach that hospitalists took to caring for patients was very different from geriatricians. The focus was certainly on trying to get a patient out of the hospital quickly, but that approach usually consisted of lot of testing, specialty referrals, and aggressive treatment, not the hallmarks of the geriatric approach to care. Our experience in Orlando reinforced the concept that in order to truly reduce overall utilization in the Medicare population, there was a need to geriatricize the hospital experience. This typically meant aggressively managing the hospitalists.

5.2   Fish Out of Water

On a very practical note, it has been my consistent observation that hospitalists tend not to fare well when they attempt to care for patients in nursing facilities. The focus in a nursing facility tends to be much more aligned with a geriatric approach to care. In this setting the care provider needs to take more of a long view of the patient. Furthermore, the nursing staff also tends to fit more into this type of care and the overall culture of a nursing facility tends to be quite different than that of an acute hospital. For this reason it should not be surprising that hospitalists are often like "fish out of water" when attempting to work in nursing homes. I have seen numerous instances where a hospitalist fails in their attempt to work in a nursing facility. While this is not an absolute, it definitely represents a very strong trend.

I would like to think that some of these observations have been changing but have trouble pointing to very many examples of such. Health systems and insurers continue to develop models of care that ultimately override the care delivered in hospitals and elsewhere, rather than actually changing the practice approach of the clinicians. Ironically, the company that ultimately bought my practice, IPC, was founded as a hospitalist company and has steadily been moving into the skilled nursing space. I have continued to hope that they will find a way to integrate the geriatric approach to care into the hospitalist model. Perhaps it is a fair question to ask if it is actually possible, based on the inherent differences between geriatricians and hospitalists. Only time will deliver the answer to that question.

Finally, I will always remember an experience I had with a geriatrician that I had hired through a recruiter. Just 1 month into his employment, he told me that he didn't like working in nursing homes. I asked him why he had done a geriatric fellowship, and he told me that it was because he couldn't get into a pulmonary one. While this is hopefully unusual, it makes a very important point. There is definitely a type of person who decides to go into geriatrics, and it is important to understand this first and foremost from a hiring perspective. Once you've gone past the point of hiring, understanding the personality and emotional nuances of a geriatrician is still important from the perspective of day-to-day management.

5.3   What Is a Geriatrician

It is also important to realize that board certification does not define a geriatrician. I have known some wonderful geriatricians who never did a geriatric fellowship and were not board certified. I have also known some geriatricians who had both credentials but didn't reflect the approach and principles that reflect most of us who practice geriatrics. At the end of the day, being a geriatrician is in ones heart.

Many geriatricians will tell you that they grew up having a close relationship with their grandparents or some other elder in their family. They might have worked in a nursing home as a teenager. It is highly unusual for a geriatrician not to have some connection to an older adult prior to making their decision to enter the field. One might ascertain certain characteristics that stem from having had this type of relationship: first of all, a heartfelt tendency to care for older people and, second, a natural tendency to be willing to listen to what they have to say. Over the years I have had the opportunity to hear fascinating stories that reflect both living history and a lifetime of experiences. This may be one of the reasons that geriatricians are known to have the highest job satisfaction among physicians. Historically, that also happens to go along with having the lowest income, but with changing demographics, that will hopefully change based on traditional supply and demand concepts.

Why does the psychological makeup of geriatricians and other geriatric healthcare providers matter? Because, if you don't understand how the clinicians caring for this population of patients think, you risk developing the wrong business approach to managing them. In fact, traditional productivity-based models of reimbursement generally do not work well with geriatricians. It's not because they are either unwilling or uninterested in working hard. It's actually the opposite. Geriatricians and geriatric healthcare providers are among some of the most dedicated and hardest-working clinicians that I have had the honor of working with. It's just that they don't want to see themselves as providing care to people as if they were widgets. Caring providers genuinely like being appreciated for being compassionate and dedicated. While making a good living certainly appeals to them, they generally prefer that aspect of their job to occur behind the scenes.

5.4   Achieving Balance

How does one balance the importance of bringing in revenue with the psychological necessity of focusing on patient care? When we first started Senior Care of Colorado, our provider contracts were essentially based on our clinicians' productivity. We did this to protect the company, but it quickly became apparent that most of our providers never really paid attention to their productivity data or revenue. The main reason was that their focus was on their patients, and I believe that they were genetically unable to switch this focus to pay attention to their actual productivity. We quickly switched to a salaried model, which garnered a very positive response.

The most important thing to recognize about clinicians who provide care to older adults is that they are hard workers. What is then critical is figuring out how to capture all of that work from a reimbursement perspective. This is what is really at the heart of all physician reimbursement and compensation issues. One must therefore devise a system that recognizes the care that the clinicians provide. Similarly, one has to make sure that the providers are accurately and completely documenting the care that they are performing. Finally, one must translate all of that work to appropriate coding and billing. If all of these elements are achieved, one has the foundation for a highly successful geriatric practice.

How does one do this from a business perspective? First, it is absolutely essential to fully understand any and all payment methodologies that a practice will be working with. Typically at the heart of a geriatric practice is fee-for-service Medicare reimbursement. There are also opportunities to work under bundled or capitated arrangements. There is no question that these types of alternative payment models will become more prominent. There is also a growing trend toward incentive-based payment models. I will go into further detail on how to operationalize these different models in another chapter. The key point here is to understand how to get providers to either accept or work within these different methods.

Fee-for-service reimbursement is traditionally known as "eat what you kill." Enough said, as this concept certainly conflicts with the moral compass of most geriatricians. Historically, most geriatricians have practiced in academic settings, where little attention was placed on their productivity. This has been changing in the last several years but has also been associated with a great amount of angst. Geriatricians working in private practice settings often receive lower compensation than their less trained colleagues. This is generally due to the expectation that they will not be as productive.

Bundled or capitated payments actually fit a geriatricians style quite well, with the caveat that if these payments are based on traditional productivity metrics, there will ultimately be pressure by the practice on the individual provider. Bundled payments for chronically ill patients actually provide a potential reimbursement alternative if the payment truly reflects the overall cost of such patients to the Medicare program.

Incentive-based payment models are the most complex. When it comes down to making a decision regarding the care of a patient, knowing that an expensive procedure might lead to lower pay is a very difficult position to put any clinician in, much less a geriatrician. Ironically, geriatricians tend to practice a much less procedurally based approach to care. They tend to refer fewer patients to specialists, hospitalize their patients less frequently, and prescribe fewer medications. This is actually the reason I went to work for Kaiser-Permanente when I started my career as a geriatrician. It made obvious sense to me that a geriatric approach to care was also a very cost-effective one. Still, there will be unique circumstances with individual patients where these issues might prove to be problematic.

5.5   The Aversion to Making Money

The other aspect of incentive-based payment models in regard to geriatricians goes back to their underlying mistrust of making money off of patients. I will not try to make sense of this response; I'm just recognizing it. Those that choose to ignore this very typical view of a geriatric clinician will ultimately have to deal with it in practice. *Most geriatricians that I have worked with have an inherent aversion to the concept that they are making money off of patients.* This really cannot be repeated too often in this chapter. The focus of a provider of care to older adults is on the provision of care, not the making of money. It's as if they have a specific gene that responds negatively to the concept of looking at a patient as a means toward an end. Their focus, as it should be, is solely on the health and well-being of the patient. This may be why I often refer to practicing geriatrics as practicing old-fashioned frontier medicine. There was a time that most doctors went into medicine because they truly wanted to help people. That's not to say that today's doctors don't want to help people. It's just that geriatricians tend to see this as their sole focus. They are the doctors that patients want to be cared for by.

5.6   Putting the Focus on Patient Care

Although we had switched to a salaried model of reimbursement at Senior Care, in order for our practice to operate successfully, we still needed to pay attention to our individual provider's productivity. We had started by developing "work value units" by which to monitor our clinicians. This gave us the opportunity to have a focal point for training our providers on proper coding. It also became a sticking point for complaints among our clinicians. Morale is an important aspect of a practice. *If you have low morale, you will ultimately have increased turnover.* Turnover of clinicians carries with it a huge cost that is often overlooked. We found that our providers didn't like the fact that their patients were money-making widgets. As I have noted in this chapter, this is a fairly common occurrence among geriatricians and geriatric nurse practitioners. Hence, we had to come up with a solution. What we ultimately did was to rename "work value units" with "patient care units."

By putting the focus on patient care, we were able to recognize all of the hard work that our clinicians provided to their patients. By training them to document the work they did, we were able to capture all of their work in order to appropriately bring in revenue for the practice. Our providers and practice thrived under this approach.

The "patient care unit" approach did not prevent us from having providers who would work 12 h a day and code for 4 h worth of work. However, it made it easier for us to demonstrate to them that they were doing so. We would have our clinicians fill out a daily diary. Upon reviewing the care that they provided for the day, we could show them that they weren't accurately capturing the care that they were providing during a day of work. This process helped us to improve the documentation and coding of some of our most caring and dedicated clinicians who might otherwise have been judged as being unproductive.

Are there geriatricians who can function and even thrive under a pure productivity-based model that is tied solely to revenue? Certainly. However, it has been my experience that this is not the norm. As the focus of clinicians who provide care to the frail elderly is the word "care," they often perceive that a production-based model doesn't put "care" first. Unfortunately, there are plenty of circumstances in today's healthcare market where this is true. Procedure-based care that has not been proven to improve quality of life is quite rampant. The physicians providing this care certainly mean well, and in fact, this is how they were trained to care for patients. It is not surprising, however, that geriatricians who practice more instinctually recognize that this is not the best approach to care, and they tend to gravitate to a "high-touch, low-tech" approach to care.

5.7   Why Go into Geriatrics?

We live in a healthcare world where young physicians and other healthcare providers are not encouraged to enter the field of geriatrics. The negative influences are myriad. Reimbursement is poor. Frail older adults and their families are often perceived as the most difficult to deal with. Caring for bed-bound, demented individuals in nursing homes will not strike most people as alluring. The people who enter this field have to want to be there. They have to be pulled into geriatrics by an inner drive to care for older people. The type of person that gravitates in this direction might be expected to be turned off by procedurally based care that focuses on revenue production. This represents a broader policy issue that we must ultimately address if we are going to positively impact the growing need for a workforce with enough clinicians to care for our rapidly expanding older population. With that said, we have to deal with the workforce that we presently have. There are still a lot of good clinicians out there, who truly want to do the right thing and provide good care for their patients.

Instead of trying to change the personality of a provider, it always struck me as prudent to focus on their inner drive and to take advantage of it. Encourage clinicians to "care" for their patients. Reward them for spending time and dealing with the multiple comorbidities and challenges that the frail elderly face. At the same time, try to find ways to encourage them to document the good work that they were doing so that they can be adequately recognized for the work they are doing.

When we live in a healthcare market where a good geriatrician with a double board certification is paid less than an internist who sees 30 patients a day, we have a problem. Fortunately, there has been some recognition of this. Medicare is encouraging innovative payment models and reimbursement reform, recognizing that the existing system does not work. Hopefully, these new approaches will recognize the unique traits of clinicians who provide care to older adults and find ways to reward them for quality geriatric care. *If a geriatric practice wishes to be financially successful, they will need to recognize these opportunities and learn how to take advantage of them.*

Going to Battle and Standing Your Ground

Geriatricians tend to be consensus builders. We generally do not like confrontation. But conflicts are inevitable. While we might wish it were not so, if you are going to be successful in business, you will be going into battle at some point along the way. The fact of the matter is that this is really the same as life. So I am going to use some of my life experiences to help make some key points that should be helpful in successfully operating a geriatrics practice.

Halfway through the 1st year of my geriatric fellowship program, I was approached by the Chief of Medicine at a managed care organization in Southern California. I had been moonlighting there since I was a 2nd-year resident, and they knew of my interest in geriatric medicine. They were ready to hire a geriatrician and develop a geriatric program. Was I interested? This was a wonderful opportunity for someone like myself. However, I was only 6 months into a 2-year fellowship program. The opportunity was right now. I could wait, but that had never been my temperament. Besides, I didn't know if the opportunity would still be there in a year and a half. There were other interesting factors. In 1989, if I were to complete my 2-year geriatric fellowship, I could immediately take the geriatric certification examination. On the other hand, if I only completed 1 year of fellowship, I would have to wait until I had 2 years of practice experience to take the exam. Of course, the end result would be the same, I would still be board certified in geriatric medicine. I had already published a paper in the Journal of the American Geriatrics Society.[1] This was definitely a crossroad for me. I would essentially be eliminating academic medicine as a career path. On the other hand, I had the opportunity to start a geriatrics program within a managed care organization.

---

[1] M Wasserman, M Levinstein, E Keller, et al. Utility of fever, white blood cells, and differential count in predicting bacterial infections in the elderly. J Am Geriatr Soc 1989;37(6):537–43.

© Springer International Publishing Switzerland 2016
M. Wasserman, *The Business of Geriatrics*, DOI 10.1007/978-3-319-28546-7_6

6.1   Weighing My Options

I weighed all of the pros and cons. The lure of getting out into the "real world" was very appealing. Having wanted to be a geriatrician since medical school, I had already been a self-learner. Every older patient I had seen as a resident was an opportunity to learn about geriatrics. In fact, the geriatric literature was scarce, making a real-world opportunity even more compelling. My decision was made. I would leave my fellowship after 1 year and join the managed care organization. I knew that it would be hard to tell my Fellowship Program Director of my decision. In 1989, the academic path was really the main one that most geriatricians were taking, and I knew they would be disappointed to lose me to the outside world. What I didn't anticipate was a senior faculty member deciding that he would do everything in his power to stop me from leaving the fellowship.

6.2   Dealing with Bullies

Before going on and sharing this story, I think it is important to identify the key learning objective. *In life and in business, we will encounter people in positions of authority who will use their position and perceived power in order to attempt to influence our decisions.* This would not be my first experience with this type of authority and it definitely would not be my last. How I dealt with it at the time definitely influenced how I would deal with these types of situations in the future.

There were several threats made to me at the time. There is no real point in rehashing each of them specifically. What is important is that I researched each and every threat. I made phone calls, and I went to the library (this was before the Internet). I discovered that there was no merit to any of the threats. I was angry, but instead of lashing out or reacting, I set up a meeting with my program director. I described the opportunity that I had, and I mentioned the threats that had been made against me. After outlining how I had discovered that all of the threats were bogus, I noted that I was prepared to retain an attorney to deal with the situation. It was at that point that the program director stopped me and told me that wouldn't be necessary. She explained that the person making the threats was used to getting his way and that she and the rest of the department were supportive of my decision. There were never any further issues about my decision. Of note, over the past 25 years, the people who were my teachers and mentors at the time have been incredibly supportive, and many have become friends and colleagues. More importantly, and this may be the most important message, is that when I had the opportunity in later years to run across the faculty member who had threatened me, I always approached him with a smile and an outstretched hand. *Never burn bridges.*

Ironically, it was only a few years later that I encountered my next similar situation. I had started a geriatric clinic in the managed care organization that I had joined after my fellowship and had taken on a multitude of new responsibilities. I realized that my ability to grow the program was being constrained by my primary care practice. As I had no real desire to care for young people (anyone under the age of 65), I went to my medical director with a request to gradually dissolve my primary care panel of patients under the age of 65. As I sat there, waiting for a response, he pulled out a piece of paper and began reading a complaint from another physician. The complaint had to do with a very challenging and difficult patient and family that our clinic had actually done a good job with. Nevertheless, this physician had perceived that there was an issue getting the patient into our clinic and had decided to write a letter of complaint.

Changing the topic is a standard method for a bully to try to throw you off guard. This method can be used by an employee or an employer. When used by someone in a position of authority, it can be particularly uncomfortable. When used by someone subordinate to you, it can be distracting. Either way, it is important to develop strategies to respond to such deflections. In the case of my medical director and his reading of the complaint letter, I calmly explained that despite there being a long wait list for our clinic, we had actually managed to get his patient into our clinic. By the way, the reason I was there was that we had a long wait list. That was because I was overextended. In fact, I had data that demonstrated that I was far and away the most productive member of my department. I had been contributing in a variety of manners and had actually garnered an award for my work. Never enter a battle unprepared. Having all of these facts at my disposal allowed me to effectively deal with the onslaught of direct challenges that I was facing.

While the medical director tried to find ways to pierce my armor, I continued to hold steady and support my position. I will never forget the feeling that I had at the end of the meeting. It was as if I had survived a 15-round heavyweight fight. But I had survived. I ultimately got what I wanted, and I hope that I earned some respect from the medical director.

6.3 Having Confidence

Those of us who enter the field of geriatrics tend to be consensus-building team players. We are not confrontational and like those around us to be happy and satisfied. When we come upon a situation where there are conflicting wants and needs, we tend to want to help everyone else achieve their goals, sometimes to the exclusion of our own desires. This type of personality can be a detriment when interacting with someone who takes a bullying or authoritative approach. In order to survive a confrontation with a bully, you must have confidence in your core beliefs. *Relying on my belief in the value of the geriatric approach to care has been instrumental in my ability to steadfastly stand my ground.*

One of the most challenging situations that I have encountered over the years relates to my actions as a nursing home medical director. As I will address in another chapter, being the medical director of a nursing home comes with a lot of conflicting issues. First and foremost, being a medical director is generally a contractual relationship. Yet, even if one is employed directly by the facility, the responsibility of a medical director to the patients (notice the use of the word patients rather than residents) in the facility is one that must reflect our Hippocratic Oath. Nevertheless, being a medical director is also a business relationship. To some degree, it may imply that we also will care for patients in the facility, and this may be a significant source of revenue for our practice. The medical directorship itself may also be a significant source of revenue.

6.4   Standing Up for Quality

What happens when, as a nursing home medical director, I become concerned about the quality of care that the facility is delivering to its residents? I have had the occasion where this has happened. It becomes my responsibility to tell the administrator that the facility cannot accept any new admissions. Clearly, this type of decision has the potential to negatively impact the revenue of the facility. The administrator might ultimately respond to my decision by canceling my contract or even reducing the number of admissions that my practice receives. What do I do under these circumstances? I have found that honesty is always the best policy. In what appears to be a continuing theme in this chapter, it is always important to have one's ducks in a row. Collecting the necessary data and arming oneself with the appropriate facts, it is almost as if we are entering a debate.

When I have encountered situations where I determine that I must not allow admissions to my nursing facility, I will tend to couch my decision in the potential ramifications of making the wrong decision. If a facility accepts admissions when it ought not to, it is risking a bad survey and, worse, negative outcomes that could have a catastrophic impact on its reputation in the community. Losing a few admissions for a few days may cause short-term financial losses but can prevent a long-term result that may be very difficult to recover from. Furthermore, the rest of the community will typically be impressed by, and respectful of, such a decision. In the end, it is always worthwhile to try to make lemonade out of lemons.

6.5   Courageous Coding

Arguably, the most frightening and potentially disastrous challenge that Senior Care of Colorado ever faced had to do with its "relationship" with the Office of Inspector General (OIG). While I will fully discuss this experience in another chapter, the story also belongs here, under the context of the need to be courageous when it comes to coding and billing in today's healthcare world. I give full credit to my business partner, Dr. Don Murphy, for recognizing and promoting this concept. As has been the continuous theme of this chapter, it comes down to whether you believe in what you are doing.

When we started Senior Care of Colorado, we knew that it was critical for us to understand Medicare's coding rules. Since potentially 100 % of our revenue would be collected based on how we followed these rules, we took it upon ourselves to become experts in them. As we became more and more knowledgeable, it became apparent to us that many physicians were fearful of a government audit and subsequently undercoded for the work that they performed. This had the unfortunate consequence of making a geriatric practice unprofitable. Fortunately, when we looked at the rules and ran the numbers, we realized that accurate coding was consistent with a successful practice. Naively, I thought that since we were geriatricians trying to provide high-quality care to our patients, we would be immune from a government audit. Boy was I wrong!

6.6 Stepping on Toes

Coming on to the geriatric healthcare scene in the Denver marketplace, some of the local nursing homes were very excited that we owned a couple of clinics. They probably perceived, albeit incorrectly, that we would be able to supply them with patients. They also understood that we were experts in geriatric medicine. Anyways, we were soon bombarded with offers to take positions as medical directors in a number of nursing facilities. What we didn't pay much attention to was that for us to be offered a position as medical director, someone would be losing a position. We are pretty sure to this day that one of those physicians was upset and contacted the OIG, claiming that we had accepted a medical director position under false pretenses.

On a very positive note, we were meticulous when it came to documenting the work that we did as medical directors, so when the investigators reviewed our time sheets and our contracts, they could find no wrongdoing. The first lesson is always to follow the rules. One year into the investigation, the government changed direction. Since they couldn't find anything wrong with our medical director relationships, they switched over to investigating our billings. This was clearly the government's sweet spot when it came to trying to intimidate physicians. In fact, as we subsequently discovered, many physicians are so afraid of this that they literally undercode in order to avoid any scrutiny. Considering how many physicians say that it is impossible to make a living seeing Medicare patients, this approach certainly does not work.

6.7 Preparing for Battle

Once we realized that the government was looking at our billing records, we had to prepare for battle. This involved hiring a law firm to provide us with guidance. We looked closely at our internal documentation and coding educational process. We conducted our own audits. There is that trend yet again! Be prepared! No matter what the circumstance, when one encounters a challenge, it's time to batten down the hatches, get organized, and know more than your opponent. I will continue the discussion of our experience with the OIG in a later chapter. Suffice it to say, our battles and challenges come to us from all directions. *Do your homework, don't be afraid, and remember that one makes their own luck!*

I have encountered many geriatricians over the years who have complained about having difficulties getting new programs enacted. Since we often are not blessed with reams of data supporting our positions, it is common for us to minimize our certainty over the potential success of programs that we believe in. In the end, we do ourselves no favors with this approach. Whether we are part of a larger organization or are making a case to a potential business partner, we must be firm in our conviction and steadfast in our willingness to stand our ground for what we believe.

As I have mentioned before, physicians are not typically trained in business concepts. Our job is to help people feel better. The traits and skills needed to compete in the marketplace are not necessarily inherent in geriatricians. On the other hand, most of the situations that I have mentioned in this chapter are not unique to physicians. They occur in all of our lives in various forms. We have interacted with bullies since we were on the playground as children. Many of us have encountered teachers who are enamored with the power they have over their students. All too often, those with low self-esteem will try to control others to make themselves feel better. There are many variations on this theme that we will all encounter in both life and the world of business. A geriatric practice is not immune to these challenges. How we respond to them will define our success.

By the Numbers

7

"No margin, no mission," the nuns running a catholic hospital used to say to my good friend, Jim Riopelle. Financial viability is arguably the single most important factor in what makes a successful business. Granted, quality and customer service are a close second, but if you can't pay the bills and keep the lights on, you can't provide any service, quality, or otherwise. Running a medical practice or even a large health system, ultimately there must be more money coming in than going out. An important starting point for achieving this goal is a reliable budget.

Putting together an unrealistic budget doesn't help you succeed, any more than not putting a budget together at all. Yet it is very common for business owners to be overly optimistic when predicting their revenue and expenses. While it seems easy to come up with positive revenue numbers, it's also very easy to forget certain expenses which add up enough to turn a profit into a loss. Inflation, increases in employee health insurance, and medical malpractice costs can all wreck havoc on a budget. Adding into this equation the political unknowns that have annually threatened to affect physician reimbursement, you almost have a game of Russian roulette.

I've often told people that I have a knack for numbers. There is no question that this is a useful skill when developing and running a business. At the same time, my knack for numbers didn't prevent me from allowing Senior Care of Colorado to accumulate nearly $1.5 million in debt in 2005. After the company had achieved sound financial footing in its first few years, I had formulated a rule. That rule was to always be in a position to shut the company down, collect all of the receivables, and be able to walk away without incurring any personal liability. In 2005, we came precariously close to crossing that line. The worst part was that we didn't see it coming. Our most important metric at the time was our monthly billed charges. We thought that if our charges were consistent, then our revenue would be as well.

While it may appear that the lifeblood of a medical practice has to do with seeing patients and billing for those visits, the unsung critical component is collecting on what you bill. The importance of this in a primary care practice is magnified by the fact that it is a high-volume, relatively low-margin operation. If your collections are

© Springer International Publishing Switzerland 2016
M. Wasserman, *The Business of Geriatrics*, DOI 10.1007/978-3-319-28546-7_7

messed up, it doesn't take long to fail. Moreover, the rules are always changing, so just because things have worked in the past doesn't mean that everything will go smoothly moving forward. This is what happened to us in 2005.

7.1   Monitor Your Billing Service

When we started Senior Care in 2001, we chose to use an outside billing service that we were familiar with and had some previous experience using. There is no question in my mind that anyone starting a medical practice should begin by using an outside billing service. The risks of getting it wrong by doing it yourself are too great. However, using an outside billing service does not mean avoiding close monitoring of the collection process. We ultimately went through two different billing services before we decided to take billing in-house. In the case of both outside billing companies, we left a significant amount of money on the table because they didn't have enough skin in the game, so to speak. The simple fact in a primary care medical practice is that after Medicare pays you 80 % of the bill, you still have to collect on the other 20 %. That often means trying to collect $6 to 20 from a patient or a secondary insurance company. That would be fine if all you did was send out the invoice with a 50 cent stamp and envelope, but the problem should be obvious. Most billing services earn anywhere from 3 to 10 % on the amount of collections they bring in. When you're trying to collect on a bill under $10, it actually may cost the billing service more to collect those last dollars than they will receive in fees. How hard do you think they'll work to collect that money?

Making matters even worse is the slow and often tedious response from Medigap insurance companies. If Medicare allowable is $100, you would hope to collect $100. The only thing you can be sure of, if you follow procedures properly, is to collect $80. Receiving the final $20 can be a challenge and often the one most overlooked. There is also a very fine line on how much one has to spend in order to collect this money. Similar to the billing service not finding it worthwhile to collect these last dollars, the practice itself has to try to limit the expense necessary to collect the maximum amount.

Ultimately, as our billings increased, it became clear to us that we could no longer afford to outsource our billing to an outside service. We decided to bring our billing in-house. This was not a task to be taken lightly. We needed to hire the necessary staff and have the appropriate software. We also needed someone who knew the ins and outs of billing and who would stay abreast of the ongoing curveballs that Medicare seemed to throw us. In some ways, this was a lose-lose proposition. If you bring billing in-house and mess it up, you're pretty much screwed. So we had to get it right. One of the key elements in getting billing right is having the proper metrics to follow so that you know that your billing department is doing their job. You also have to make sure that the cost of your billing department doesn't exceed the fees that you were paying to an outside service, although you must also factor in the percentage of billed charges that are actually collected. This is the piece that a lot of people miss when making this decision. If you are paying 3 % but only collecting 80 % of billed charges, that is not as good as having a 6 % administrative expense in order to collect 95 % of charges.

7.2   Taking Billing In-House

Setting up a billing department means paying attention to a variety of details. Since a geriatric practice is highly dependent on Medicare claims, this has to be done right. Since Medicare only pays 80 % of allowable charges, the Medigap claims take on significant importance. As mentioned before, this is actually one of the most problematic and often time-consuming aspects of billing. On a positive note, Medicare will pay you within 10 business days if you submit your claim electronically.

What happened to us in 2005? In some ways, we had become complacent. Over the first 4 years of the practice, our revenue had been gradually increasing every year. We had annual challenges, often related to changes in reimbursement for specific codes or new rules. We had navigated these changes pretty well and were confident in our ability to do so. We had our own billing department and things seemed to be going well. However, the biggest risk of doing billing yourself comes from the chance that you develop glitches in your system. This is what happened to us in 2005. We had a systemic problem in our billing system and procedures that led to a number of Medicare claims not being paid. Since our main metric at the time was looking at how much we were billing out each month, we didn't initially notice that our collections were not matching up. The fact that this happened at the beginning of the year, when claims are not always paid due to patient deductibles, made it more difficult for us to notice initially. It doesn't take long for a shortfall to pile up.

Our "CFO" at the time was someone who had been with us for some time, and our practice had outgrown their capabilities. Unfortunately, we did not realize this initially. They didn't know how to ask for help or admit that they were in over their head. Finally, as we approached the limit of our line of credit, we sat down and literally walked through the life of a Medicare claim, examining all of our data. In performance improvement language, we performed a root cause analysis. Using this process we finally figured out that we had an unusual number of claims being kicked back and discovered where the problem was.

On a positive note, Medicare gives you 2 years to file, or in this case refile, a claim. The solution was to get the claims done properly and the money that we should have received would finally come in. There were multiple lessons from this experience. The first one was to obtain the highest line of credit that you can. When we started our practice, we had a $500,000 line of credit. Once we had completely paid off the line of credit and our cash flow was good, we went to the bank to increase our credit line. This is a very important point. *Banks will only increase your line of credit when you don't need it!* That is the time to ask, which we had done. If we hadn't had the higher line of credit, we would have been unable to withstand this incident. The other very important lesson was to track collections in addition to actual billings. This incident led us to develop a new spreadsheet that monitored our percentage of collections every week compared to the week the claims were filed. We thus knew that 4 weeks from filing claims, we should expect to have collected 60 %, 8 weeks 70 %, 12 weeks 80 %, and so on and so forth. *The margins for a primary care medical practice are thin, and not collecting just 5 % can be enough to kill a practice.* Cash flow is also important, and knowing how long it takes to collect will give you a better handle on what cash flow to expect. You can't pay bills with money in "accounts receivable."

There is a final aspect of collections that is really hard for a geriatric practice, that is, having to collect from your patients. Making a decision to send a patient to a collection service is one of the most difficult decisions a physician owner has to make. We developed a procedure for doing this that began with one of our billing staff contacting the patient or family and ended with one of the owners making a decision on whether to send the patient to collections. We took into account the patient's circumstances and tried to do the right thing. I don't know what the right approach is to this issue, and every practice needs to figure this out themselves.

7.3   Understanding Coding

While maximizing collections are critical to the success of a practice, if the coding itself is not appropriate, you may be dead before you even get out of the gate. Knowing the most common billing codes that a practice will utilize is one of the most important factors in developing a successful medical practice. One must not only know what the codes are but thoroughly understand each code and what they mean from a workflow perspective. *The biggest epiphany that we had as a practice was the understanding of time-based coding.* There were a few reasons that this was important, but first and foremost was being able to identify practice inefficiencies. *Simply put, if someone is working for 10 h and billing out for only four hours, there is a problem.* Not surprisingly, this may be one of the single most important determiners in the success, or lack thereof, of a medical practice. That is an important topic that I'll save for a later chapter. It's time to get back to the concept of budgeting!

7.4   Initiating a Budget

As I said at the onset of this chapter, all businesses should have a budget. It is common sense and good business practice. So, prior to founding Senior Care of Colorado, I prepared a budget. We were taking over existing clinics, so we had financial data from the preceding years. In many ways, this was very fortunate. As my daughter recently told me about her experience opening a restaurant, "you don't know what you don't know." What this means is that prior to starting any business, one needs to make a list of every possible expense, no matter how small or inconsequential it may seem. All expenses ultimately add up.

The other half of putting together a budget is predicting revenue. In this regard, running a geriatrics practice is relatively straightforward, or so it might seem. When we co-founded Senior Care of Colorado, we put together a budget based on the previous year's "Medicare allowable." What we failed to be aware of at the time was that the congress had enacted the Medicare Sustainable Growth Rate (SGR) formula in 1997, and in 2002, there was a 4.8 % cut to physician reimbursement.

Medicare also pays physicians differently depending on the place of service. A nursing home is different from a clinic visit. In fact, in 2002, reimbursement for patients in the category of skilled nursing care went down 15 %. On the other hand, for patients who were in custodial care, we saw our reimbursement increase! One could be providing the same service to two patients in the same room in a nursing facility, but the reimbursement would be significantly different depending on how they were categorized. That was the nursing home setting, and that was how the government set its payment rates that year.

When we started Senior Care of Colorado, assisted living facilities were considered "domiciliaries," and the reimbursement in this setting was abysmal. Nevertheless, older adults living in assisted living facilities are among the most vulnerable members of our society. My business partner, Dr. Don Murphy, saw this as an important niche that required improved access to care. We decided that we could make do with the inadequate reimbursement if we at least had some significant volume in such facilities. Hence, we embarked on a plan to have our providers visit as many of these facilities as possible. Fortunately, as luck would have it, through the extraordinary lobbying efforts of the American Medical Directors Association (AMDA) and the American Academy of Home Care Physicians, the reimbursement for caring for patients in assisted living facilities and in their own homes increased dramatically over the next couple of years. This allowed us to further focus on this needy population.

7.5 Drilling Down on Revenue Production

It is critical to look at all facets of revenue production when putting together the revenue portion of a budget. This literally means drilling down by provider the expected workflow on a daily, and ultimately annual, basis. For a geriatrics practice, this means looking at all service locations, the amount of time spent in each one, and the litany of codes that will be billed. One has to also have a full grasp of appropriate coding. This is important on multiple levels. A practice has to be on the lookout for providers who code inappropriately in either direction. As previously noted, a physician who codes 4 h worth of work during a 10 h work day is doing everyone a disservice. Similarly, a provider who codes for 26 h worth of work during a 10 h work day is putting the practice at risk. Fortunately, the E&M coding system, with all of its negative aspects and challenging rules, actually allows for good time approximations for each code that is billed. In fact, because true time-based billing actually brings in somewhat less revenue than what could be billed for by strict adherence to the E&M coding rules, the opportunity for fairly conservative budgeting exists.

Budgeting revenue production by provider has a number of benefits. It provides a metric by which to evaluate and monitor each provider. This allows the practice to monitor trends and identify potential issues. This actually happened on a number of occasions at Senior Care, especially during some periods of time where we were being intensively audited by the government or another payor. Clinicians, despite fairly intensive training on appropriate coding, would intermittently become more cautious. This caution would often lead to undercoding, a process with potentially disastrous implications. Having daily, weekly, and monthly expectations for coding provides an excellent means for monitoring such variations.

7.6   The Importance of Insurance Mix

When budgeting revenue in a medical practice, the other important factor is the insurance mix. Clearly, basing everything on Medicare allowable is the starting point, but most practices do not have 100 % of their patients on straight Medicare. Clearly, there is some greater simplicity in a pure geriatric practice, but even our practice had a number of payors. Starting with Medicare, you then break patients down by those that do not have a supplemental insurer. For these patients, you must collect the additional 20 % from the patient.

Most practices will also have a percentage of patients who are also on Medicaid. These patients are called "dually eligible." Historically, this population has been highly problematic, insofar as many states paid very little of the additional 20 %. In fact, in our practice, the cost of billing for the additional amount, while required by law, exceeded what we were paid! With attempts to bring parity to Medicaid coverage, this may be changing, but definitely needs to be reevaluated on an annual basis. Furthermore, this population is in the cross-hairs of numerous attempts to affect change in the healthcare marketplace, as they tend to be among the highest utilizers of Medicare services.

Next, you get to the Medicare beneficiaries who carry Medigap coverage. As noted earlier in this chapter, collecting the 20 % on these patients can also be challenging. It is critical that a practice monitor the success of collecting from Medigap insurers and constantly be on the lookout for any patterns of denials or delayed payments.

Once traditional Medicare fee-for-service is accounted for, one gets to the Medicare Advantage programs. There are a number of ways that a practice may get paid by these programs. First is a modified fee-for-service payment. There are some insurers that will actually pay more than 100 % of what Medicare allows. Negotiating a contract with these insurers requires some acumen regarding knowledge of the marketplace, as well as historical data in regard to a practice's overall costs and utilization. A well-performing geriatrics practice can actually provide improved profitability to a Medicare Advantage program, giving added leverage to receiving a higher fee-for-service payment. On the other hand, there are also opportunities to achieve additional income through "shared-savings" programs. At Senior Care, due to our geriatric approach to care, we typically received some additional bonuses via shared-savings programs.

7.7   Co-pays

One of the most misunderstood aspects of having patients who belong to a Medicare Advantage plan has to do with co-payments. Patients tend to believe that co-payments are additional payments to their doctor. In fact, *the co-pay is assumed by the insurance company to have been paid to the practice and therefore is deducted from the actual reimbursement.* It thus becomes absolutely essential for the practice to collect co-payments. I have seen situations in a practice where a provider tells the patient that they don't have to pay the co-pay due to perceived financial hardship. While there may be situations that this could occur, it means that visit will not be paid in full. The only people who should make this type of decision are the owners of the practice. If an employed or staff physician makes this determination, they should be offered the opportunity to have the amount deducted from their own paycheck. I hate to sound harsh on issues like this, but these can be very important issues to a practice, especially if the practice cares for a significant number of Medicare Advantage patients.

Another method of payment through Medicare Advantage plans is to be capitated. This generally means receiving a set payment per member per month, or pmpm. This has a number of budgeting advantages, in particular, knowing your monthly revenue in advance and having a stable cash flow for the practice. The operational challenge with capitated payments is making sure that ultimately they are at least equal to what you would have earned with fee-for-service reimbursement. The caveat to this is that you will save on the billing and collection costs. *Doing the mathematical analysis to determine the utility of a capitated contract is fairly straightforward.* You must estimate the average number of annual visits the patients will make and the average code that the practice typically bills for. That will put you in the ballpark. Then compare what your typical reimbursement would have been for the same population and ultimately what your collections and cost of billing would average.

7.8   Bonus and Incentive Opportunities

There are a growing number of opportunities for bonuses in today's healthcare marketplace. With Medicare these tend to revolve around meeting certain quality measure metrics. At the same time, there are opportunities for penalties for not meeting these metrics. One of the important questions that should always be asked is the cost of obtaining and documenting the metrics in the first place. Sometimes the cost exceeds the bonuses and isn't as great as the penalty. With that said, one needs to take the long view and determine if the initial cost to set up a system to collect the necessary metrics declines over time. Under this scenario, one must consider this process to be an initial investment. When Medicare began with their PQRS program, we actually held back during the first year, as we perceived the cost of implementation to far exceed the financial benefits. As the program became more developed, and we learned ways to efficiently document the necessary metrics, we got fully on board with the program. *You cannot enter a quality measure program with your eyes closed!*

One of the most challenging decisions to be made in today's market has to do with electronic medical records. The bottom line is that you've got to do it. We will cover the financial, operational, and philosophical implications of this decision in another chapter.

As noted, the concept of "shared-savings" programs has been around for a number of years, and with increased pressure on value-based payment, we are sure to see this trend continue. Some of these programs will be tied to actual "savings," so there will be comparisons to specific types of expenditures. On the other hand, some of these will occur in the form of bonuses that are tied to certain utilization metrics such as hospital days per thousand. There are huge opportunities for geriatricians when it comes to this type of additional income. The importance of this is such that we will dedicate a chapter to discussing this.

When we started Senior Care in 2001, we looked around for all sources of income. As geriatricians there are actually additional opportunities available to enhance the revenue stream of a practice. The first and most common is to become a medical director of a nursing home. While I will cover this process in another chapter, it is important to note that from a budgetary perspective, it is important to compare this revenue to patient billings when it comes to the impact on an individual provider. While this looks on the surface to be additional income, if it leads to a decrease in billings, the net result could be negative.

Similarly, during the first couple years of building our practice, we were approached by a number of pharmaceutical companies to become speakers for the use of various drugs that were pertinent to the older population. Keeping in mind that these speaking fees are public knowledge today, this is additional revenue. There are a lot of philosophical issues regarding revenue such as this, but in the case of our practice, as an owner, we put this additional income into the practice in order to help it succeed in its early years.

7.9   Breaking Down Revenue Details

Finally, it is useful to break down the practices income by source, so that this can be monitored over time. This is useful strategically, if one finds that particular areas are more profitable than others, then decisions regarding growth can be influenced by this information. In the case of our practice, it became clear that nursing home revenue had the greatest margin initially, so it wasn't a surprise that our practice gravitated to having this as its largest revenue source. With that in mind, be cautious of looking only at revenue numbers. The expenses, or overhead, are just as critical. Furthermore, there are often costs that cannot be captured, such as a far greater number of phone calls in the middle of the night regarding nursing home residents compared to clinic patients. There is ultimately a cost to this that must be factored in. We will cover this in great detail when we discuss nursing home care.

While nursing home billings were the largest source of revenue for our practice, with the advent of improved payment for patient care in assisted living facilities, over the next several years, this became another significant source of income. One of the useful metrics that we began reporting was the amount of charges and collections by facility. *The critical aspect of this was that collections did not necessarily follow charges.* For example, a facility that was mostly private pay had residents with both Medicare and a Medigap carrier, so the collections in these facilities would run close to 95 % of Medicare allowable. On the other hand, in facilities with a high proportion of Medicaid residents, the collections would run closer to 85 %. *It's not just about how many patients you see in an hour. You still have to collect!*

Another advantage to breaking down charges by facility is the ability to look for trends. While the providers themselves may notice trends, numbers don't lie. A decline in charges may relate to a decrease in admissions to a particular facility. We had a situation once where a competing group made a deal with a facility to get all of the new admissions. While I will save a discussion of this dynamic for another chapter, needless to say, our charges dropped pretty quickly at that facility. Provider coding and billing habits are not necessarily static; they can fluctuate at times. If a provider is slowing down, or perhaps is getting nervous about how to code because of something they heard or read in the newspaper, one may also see a decline in total charges. In this case, knowing the charge per visit becomes important. *Undercoding is one of the most damaging things to hit a medical practice and requires great vigilance and then education in order to correct it.*

7.10   Expenses Matter

Once one has all of the revenue sources accounted for in their budget, it is time to tackle the expenses! This is the most complex area for budgeting in many ways, yet, once you account for everything, it can be the most simple. Revenue may vary, but expenses are generally pretty stable. You just have to know what they are! In our case, we had acquired the assets of an existing practice that already had historical profit and loss statements. This is the easiest way to start, but the concepts are still the same. Review all of the ongoing expenses that you expect to have. I also developed a very important habit. Always overestimate your expenses!

Let's go down the key expense areas for a medical practice, starting with payroll. The reason I like to start with reviewing payroll expenses is multifold. First, when you talk about employee compensation, everyone focuses on salary. Unfortunately, this only covers a portion of the actual payroll expense. Additional benefits are very important, especially if they include health insurance, which has definitely continued to drive up employee benefit costs. FICA is something that must be taken into account, as the employer is responsible for an equal contribution to social security and Medicare. There are also worker's compensation payments. If one is in a competitive market, items like a 401 K come into play as well. All of these factors can easily add 20–30 % to an employee's salary.

Malpractice insurance is an obvious expense that affects each individual physician's overall cost. One also has to pay attention to how they address malpractice coverage if that physician leaves the practice. Today, most physicians carry "claims-made" insurance. Because the physician, and hence the practice, is still liable if a claim is made after the physician has left the practice, it is critical that "tail coverage" is either bought or provided when a physician leaves the practice.

Health insurance has and will continue to be a very important line item in the expense budget. When wages were frozen during World War II, providing health insurance as an employee benefit began to take hold. Today's increasingly costly health insurance marketplace has made this a key issue. Most practices will pay a portion of their employee's health insurance, and that portion has tended to decline with the rapid increases in health insurance premiums. This becomes an important issue to look at every year, not only for fiscal purposes but for employee morale. Changing health insurance options can be a traumatic event for one's employees, so a lot of planning needs to go into decisions made regarding this issue.

Instead of going through the entire list of typical expense items in this chapter, I have included a sample budget in a table for reference. *Don't forget any expense line items in your budget!*

Income	
Patient revenue	Billing collections
	Co-pays
	Medical record fees
	PQRS
	Capitated revenue
	Shared savings
Medical director revenue	NH medical director revenue
	Other medical director revenue
Non-patient revenue	Honorarium
	Expert witness revenue
	Other revenue
Expenses	
Personnel	Physicians
	Nonphysician providers
	Clinical staff
	Administrative staff
Employee benefits	Health insurance
	Dental insurance
	Vision insurance
	Life insurance
	Long-term disability
	Short-term disability
	401 K match
Education	Licenses
	Dues
	Subscriptions
	CME
Credentialing	Credentialing
Other personnel expenses	Worker's compensation
	Payroll service charge
	Recruiting expense
	Payroll taxes
Rent	Facility rent

Office expenses	Building repairs
	Computer repairs
	Equipment repairs
	Maintenance
Utilities	Infectious waste
	Utilities
Telecommunications	Internet/telephone
	Answering service
	Cellular phones
Equipment	Computer
	Office
Supplies	Medical supplies
	Office supplies
	Marketing supplies
Other expenses	Printing
	Postage
	Water
	Medical record copying
Outside services	Laundry and uniforms
	Courier service
	Shredding service
	Other
Office expenses	
General and administrative	Malpractice insurance
	Auto insurance
	Other insurance
Travel and entertainment	Meals
	Entertainment
	Airfare
	Lodging
	Car rental
Professional fees	Accounting
	Legal fees
	Consulting
Miscellaneous	Contributions
	Dues
	Gifts
	Service charges
	Lock box fees
	Misc
	Loan interest
Taxes	Property taxes
Amortization and depreciation	

Swimming with the Sharks

8

Physicians, by the very nature of their profession, want to help people. It is generally anathema to think first about taking care of themselves. Businesses, by their very nature, must look out for themselves first. This sets up a dichotomy that has challenged doctors for an eternity. We swim along in our practice, focusing on caring for our patients. We also have to make a living, so first we tend to meld our business practices with the approach to care that we learned in medical school and residency. This can be very challenging for geriatricians, who often believe that the geriatric approach to care is not conducive to adequate revenue production. Even for those of us who have managed to make this work, the deep dark waters of the rest of the healthcare world lurk outside our office.

Part of being in the business of delivering geriatric care is dealing with all of the outside forces around us. The world of managed care, or whatever new names are given to various risk-sharing arrangements that will abound in the future, can easily be likened to swimming with the sharks. I actually say this with the utmost respect for this approach, as I actually began my career out of my fellowship as a firm believer that a managed care model was the future of geriatric care. Ironically, 25 years later, I still believe this to be the case!

8.1 Doing the Right Thing

As I have stated before, geriatrics is about quality of life and function. Good geriatric care tends to be a very high-touch and low-tech approach to care. Geriatricians view hospitals as dangerous places and do not like to have their patients undergo procedures. Hospitals and procedures are expensive, so avoiding them can save lots of money. I love to tell my patients that I have discontinued more medications in my career than I have prescribed. The cost of pharmaceuticals is an annually growing number. It doesn't take long to realize that a geriatric approach to care can and should be very cost-effective. It was with this in mind that I embarked upon my career by joining a large group model HMO right out of my geriatric fellowship.

© Springer International Publishing Switzerland 2016
M. Wasserman, *The Business of Geriatrics*, DOI 10.1007/978-3-319-28546-7_8

A managed care company should understand that investing in an approach that ultimately reduces hospitalization and procedures is bound to be financially successful. This concept made absolute sense to me over 25 years ago. To this day, I continue to make this the hallmark of my approach to geriatric care modeling. What continues to frustrate me is the general lack of understanding that the healthcare industry has tended to have with this theory. That may be changing, but it would still be unwise to ignore the past.

One of my first big disagreements with the managed care organization that I began my career with was when they decided to increase the co-pay for office visits for Medicare beneficiaries. I was quite upset by this. It seemed so obvious to me that our goal was to see the frail elderly more frequently, in order to prevent health problems and avoid unnecessary hospitalizations. Office co-pays could be an impediment to these visits. It seemed to make sense that we should be encouraging patients to be seen, not discouraging them from making an appointment. Over the years, I have seen this mistake repeated many times by many managed care companies. The short-term need for revenue will often win out over the long-term impact of reduced office visits. The irony of the co-pay situation in relation to a private medical practice is that it solely benefits the insurance company, because the co-pay is deducted from the physician's reimbursement. So, the insurance company makes more money, the physician doesn't make any more, and in fact is at risk for making less because the patient is discouraged from being seen. The end result does not improve care nor does it save money.

8.2 Playing Hardball

When we started Senior Care of Colorado, it turned out that we were the most robust geriatric practice in Denver and had the ability to provide coverage at a number of skilled nursing facilities. Knowing this, when it came time to sign a contract with our local managed care company to provide skilled nursing coverage, we held out for 125 % of Medicare allowable! In one of our most "successful" negotiating stances ever, we actually stared down a large HMO and they caved at the last moment. We had that contract for the next couple of years, until such time that they dropped us like a rock and replaced us with another group that one of their medical directors had actually started on the side! There is a lesson in this. Be careful not only when swimming with the sharks, but when you decide to take them on in battle. *Short-term victories do not always translate into long-term wins.* "Winning" the initial negotiation ultimately proved harmful to our business a couple of years later. It took us a few more years to get that business back, which we ultimately did by providing better service in the marketplace.

When looking back at our skilled nursing coverage negotiations, we missed an incredible opportunity. We were in a position of strength and we took advantage of it to secure higher reimbursement. In retrospect, we could have used that position to improve our relationship by offering better service and solidifying a longer-term relationship with the managed care entity. As a geriatric service provider, we knew that the patients we cared for would have lower lengths of stay and reduced rehospitalizations. *Instead of promoting our positive outcomes and quality, however, we got too focused on the monetary aspect of things and missed a great opportunity.*

Negotiating with a managed care payor can be a very daunting process. A small practice will generally have no leverage and will be forced either to accept the contract terms or not accept patients that belong to that HMO. Larger practices have a little more clout, depending on the rest of the market. Size does matter when it comes to negotiating contract terms. One of the things that a geriatric practice does have when it comes to leverage is its patients. Again, the larger the practice, the more the patients, which means more leverage. When we started Senior Care of Colorado, we sat down with our local HMO (the same one that we stared down with our SNF negotiations) and offered to work with them on enlisting our patients to join their HMO. Ironically, at the time, we thought that this was going to be the best approach for our practice to achieve profitability. What we ultimately found was that only a quarter of our patients were willing to switch from fee-for-service to an HMO. We had to adjust our approach, which we did. Nevertheless, the HMO was more willing to work with us on our contract due to our willingness to work with them.

8.3   Knowledge Is Leverage

It should be clear that one of the greatest leverage points that we have with a managed care payor is our patients. The reason for this is simple, money. The HMO gets a significant amount of money every month for every patient that signs up with them. The next leverage point that geriatricians have is our approach to care. While this is obvious to us, it may not be as obvious to the HMO. We must do a good job of convincing the HMO that our approach to care is cost-effective. They need to believe that the way we care for their members will lower their expenditures. Experience matters here, as does data. Over time, it is very important to be aware of the key data points that you can use when having any new negotiations. If you know that your specialty utilization is low, or that your hospital admission rate is low, these are valuable tools. The HMO doesn't mind making money off of your practice, and they're probably not going to tell you how much they're making! You need to tell them. This requires knowledge of the HMO's financial structure.

The advent of accountable care organizations will also provide many opportunities for geriatric providers to have a positive impact on the overall cost of care to Medicare beneficiaries. In fact, it is in this space that we may have our greatest opportunity. Not only is there a reasonable amount of data, but there is actually plenty of real-world experience to support this concept. So why isn't our field growing in leaps and bounds? Why aren't ACOs running to hire as many geriatricians as possible? Why isn't the geriatric approach to care expanding like the big bang?

I believe that the reason involves both what I call "institutional arrogance" and the need to hold on to what existing businesses are comfortable with. Large organizations tend to believe that they must know everything. That's why they're so big and successful after all, isn't it? Healthcare systems are also entrenched in decades of patterns. These patterns are responsible for significant flows of revenue. Let's face it; hospitals do not make money (yet) if they are empty. Cath labs do not bring in revenue if there are no patients. Specialists do not make a living if they are sitting at their desks with nothing to do (again, yet). Furthermore, we physicians are creatures of habit. We have been trained to aggressively treat diabetes, despite recent literature that suggests otherwise in older adults. We have been trained to aggressively treat hypertension, despite a lack of literature in those over the age of 85. We have been trained to diagnose, treat, and cure, when frail elderly are more concerned about quality of life and function. Changing physician behavior is not something that will happen overnight. It is a process. Fortunately, geriatricians are already attuned to this approach to care. Unfortunately, there are not a lot of us out there. Juxtapose that with the size, clout, arrogance, and inertia of hospitals and insurance companies and you have the challenging task of trying to move an immoveable rock.

Fortunately for us, the immoveable rock is unsustainable. Healthcare costs have risen to a degree that has pushed both businesses and individuals to start crying uncle. Medicare is a huge component of the federal budget. With the increasing number of baby boomers turning 65, and the rapid growth in the over 85 population, society has begun to understand that the status quo is unacceptable. For all of its imperfections, the Affordable Care Act shifted the immoveable rock and began to push it out of its hole. A number of components of the ACA, as well as market pressures on each facet of the healthcare industrial complex, have created opportunities for geriatricians.

8.4 Crossroads

Healthcare is at a crossroads. Many of the ACOs are owned and operated by hospital systems. There is a realization that they might actually benefit financially if their beds are empty. They realize that it might be ok to pay a specialist to do nothing. Managed care companies are finally grappling with these same issues. Historically, so long as they made their profit margin, it didn't really matter how the money was spent. The ACA put some constraints on those margins, and now it really matters what happens in regard to the care that patients receive. With all of these changes, there will be opportunities for geriatricians, but they must be ready and prepared to take them! It will be necessary for us to have data readily available to support our approach and models of care. We cannot be timid, as there will be others trying to access the up-front dollars that run a healthcare system. *It will be critical to draw a line and make the case for our approach to be delivered up front in order to save money and resources down the line.*

Disease management companies are one of the most interesting roadblocks that have gotten in the way of the geriatric approach and model of care. Back in the mid-1990s, Oxford Health was the darling of Wall Street. As a Medicare HMO, they had gone the route of multiple disease management programs. They had programs for heart failure, heart disease, diabetes, etc. The contractors for these programs each boasted that they were saving millions of dollars for Oxford Health. The stock kept going up, until 1 day, Oxford reported its earnings. They were losing millions of dollars. How could this be? The simple reason is obvious. Frail older adults tend to have multiple chronic illnesses. Having a single and separate disease management program for each problem makes no sense. The proper solution, in my opinion, is the geriatric approach and model of care. Alas, at the time, we geriatricians were not in a place, did not have the data, and definitely did not have the capital to approach the Oxford Healths of the world. This leads to one of my favorite stories.

8.5 Being Too Brash

I was President of GeriMed of America and we approached one of the largest insurers in the country about developing a geriatric care coordination program. Being the brash young geriatrician that I was at the time, I basically came out and said that separate disease management programs were worthless. While I was right, I didn't realize that the VP of the insurer that we were meeting with was the architect of their companies' disease management programs. They were his baby. I had insulted him. In the middle of our discussion, he stood up and walked out of the room. End of deal. I was devastated. Lesson learned, *just because you're right, doesn't mean you have to tell anybody.*

Years later, in the middle of a major negotiation that would have a profound impact on my future, I was able to utilize the same technique. We were at an impasse in negotiations. The other side had actually made an error in their calculations that I had not sorted out. I got up and walked out of the room. They wanted to make the deal, and ultimately it worked out. By the way, this method does not have a guaranteed outcome. Use it at your own risk!

In order for geriatricians to successfully swim with the sharks, we must be able to speak their language. We must understand their techniques. We have to read their playbook. We don't have to become them. We don't have to forgo our inherent desire to put our patients first. We just need to be aware of the various market forces that surround us. Ironically, many of the opportunities that we have exist because of those very market forces. The same entities that historically have taken advantage of us will actually need us in order to be successful. We cannot provide these services for free. We must ask for accountability and respect. Again, these are not traits that we typically have. Fortunately, as I have noted before, if we can take care of frail older adults, we can learn how to survive in the depths of the deepest healthcare ocean.

Me and the OIG

9

I'll never forget the first time that I got word that federal agents wearing guns were interviewing administrators of some of the nursing homes where we were medical directors, and thus began my very up close and personal experience with being a target of the federal government. When we decided to start Senior Care of Colorado, I was warned that one of the risks of private practice was a government audit. I was undaunted, telling people that what we did as geriatricians was like motherhood and apple pie. Why would the government pick us as a target? We were doing necessary work that no one else wanted to do. Boy, was I wrong!

When we started Senior Care of Colorado, a number of the nursing homes in Denver decided that they were interested in us becoming medical directors of their facilities. I admit to being somewhat naive at the time. We were a group of geriatricians and were definitely skilled in being nursing home medical directors. In fact, I had first become a nursing home medical director several years earlier when a local nursing home was struggling to get patients due to perceived quality issues. I had helped turn that nursing home around in my capacity as a very active medical director, and thus began my relationship with nursing homes. While I will talk more about nursing homes specifically in the next chapter, I'll start the story here as a segue into our experience with the government.

9.1 An Opportunity Knocks

Sometime after moving to Denver to open up a hospital-based seniors' clinic with GeriMed, I was approached by a local nursing home that had fallen on hard times. They were not getting admissions from the local hospitals due to perceived quality issues. I was a geriatrician with experience in nursing home care. One of my roles when I was with Kaiser was to monitor the nursing facilities that our patients were at. I realized that I had a new opportunity to help improve the care of patients in the facility that approached me. At the same time, I realized that I had a business opportunity and I wanted to make the most of it. I essentially entered my first

© Springer International Publishing Switzerland 2016
M. Wasserman, *The Business of Geriatrics*, DOI 10.1007/978-3-319-28546-7_9

contract-related negotiation. I had something that this nursing home wanted. I had experience. I also had patients that might end up in the facility if I felt that they provided good care. This is always the catch—22 for nursing homes and medical directors. If you have a private practice, there might be the perception that you are getting paid to send your patients there. I will come back to this later.

I began my negotiation with a proposal that I would spend 6 h a week in the facility working as a medical director. This would entail reviewing the charts and rounding regularly on the skilled nursing unit with the nurses to review ongoing cases. It would include participating in all quality and safety meetings. I would be very active and be available for any problems or questions that might arise in the facility. This was unheard of at the time in the nursing home industry in Denver. In fact, it was common for a nursing home medical director at the time to spend 1–2 h a month in a facility. Their primary role was to sign forms that required a medical director's signature and perhaps sit in on one to two meetings. For this, many medical directors received $1000 a month. I proposed that I would be paid $200 per hour for my time. This was a $5,000 per month arrangement. Would they accept my proposal? To their credit, they did accept it and within 6 months, the facility was doing much better. They were getting admissions again from the local hospitals and their quality had improved significantly. Over time, I actually was able to reduce the amount of time I spent at the facility, and thus reduce my monthly reimbursement.

9.2   Fair Market Value

My role in improving the care at that nursing home was important on many levels. First of all, I had essentially set a "fair market value" for my services. Secondly, I had demonstrated the actual value of those same services. This would be important in the coming years. At the same time, it would also probably serve to make us a target for government auditors who were not used to the type of medical direction that we ascribed to. In fact, the government was actually looking to investigate medical director relationships that didn't pass muster. However, the type of relationships that the government was looking for were ones where money was exchanged but no services were provided. Fast forward several years to after the founding of Senior Care of Colorado. We were a practice of geriatricians. We worked out of two large clinics, which meant that we had a large group of patients that were at high risk for hospitalization and subsequent need for skilled nursing care. In retrospect, it is likely that a number of nursing homes perceived an opportunity to enrich their patient base by bringing on our physicians as medical directors of their facilities. At the same time, we saw an opportunity to improve the care being delivered in those facilities. Our approach to nursing home medical direction drew from my previous experiences. Our contracts typically called for at least 10 h a month of active medical director time. We got paid approximately $200 per hour for this role.

A number of nursing homes came to us and we were flattered by the interest. We accepted a number of the offers. We were naive in not recognizing that for us to be offered medical director opportunities, existing medical directors were being let go.

A number of them got upset and actually threatened their facilities. Some of the offers were withdrawn. It wasn't long after this occurred that we first got word that some nursing home administrators were being interviewed by federal agents wearing guns. The best that we could surmise was that one of the medical directors that we had displaced had contacted the OIG (Office of Inspector General) and complained that we were getting some kind of deal to become medical directors in return for admissions. This had absolutely never been the case, but *perception is always what matters*.

One of the really good habits that I had gotten into as a medical director was thoroughly documenting the time that I spent every month in my role. This was critical on multiple fronts, but in particular, it needed to line up with our monthly invoice to the facility for our services. Every minute of our time was accounted for. In fact, we had a standard medical director timesheet that allowed our physicians to document the time they spent each month. Every one of our physicians was required to fill out a form monthly, and that form was tied to the invoice that we sent to the nursing facility.

9.3   Listen to Legal Counsel

The first thing that we did when we heard that we were being investigated was to retain legal counsel. This was important and wise on multiple fronts. First, we were very much out of our league when it came to being investigated by the federal government. There are a lot of rules to follow, and our attorneys were quick to let us know what those rules were. First of all, it was important that all communication regarding the investigation go through our attorneys. This was critical in order to maintain the confidentiality of attorney-client privilege. It was important that we not have random conversations about the investigation, as these conversations could be used if a case was ever brought against us. It was also important that we notify our staff and clinicians about the investigation. The first reason was to give them instructions as to what to do if they were approached by federal agents. We needed to be able to respond quickly if this occurred.

Another aspect of notifying our clinicians was internal damage control. We didn't want any rumors to start, and we wanted everyone to know that we had everything under control. In fact, we were very confident that we had nothing to worry about. Our record keeping had been meticulous, and all we had done was provide a quality service to nursing facilities. A full year of investigation passed by without being notified of any specific problems or findings. Unfortunately, as we learned, the government doesn't like to feel like it has wasted its time. Phase two was about to commence.

We next received a subpoena requesting charts from a couple of days of nursing home visits. Since the government had been unable to find anything wrong with our medical director relationships, it went on to look at our billing records. From a cynical perspective I would tell people that they couldn't figure out how we were profitable, so they must have assumed that we were cheating. The truth was probably that they just wouldn't let go of the investigation and billing records were the logical next step. At first I wondered what they were looking at and why they had targeted the couple of days of billing records for myself and one of our other physicians. The answer became obvious very quickly. They saw that I was billing for about 45 visits per day under my provider number. They assumed that I was doing "gang visits" in the nursing home. The concept of "gang visits" was one well known to government auditors, where a physician would come to a nursing home late at night, go into the back room, and write notes of 40–50 patients without ever seeing them. Even if a physician had seen the patients, it would be difficult to perform reasonable visits on this many nursing home patients in 1 day, unless one spent 14 h in the facility and performed relatively short visits. So, what was going on?

9.4   Knowing the Rules

What the government investigators didn't understand was the concept of "incident-to" visits. A this point in time, it was still possible for a physician and nurse practitioner (or physician assistant) to see patients together at the nursing home, provided that they were on the unit together at the same time. This allowed the physician to bill for all of the visits under their provider number, thus receiving 100 % of Medicare allowable. Without "incident-to" billing, the nurse practitioners would have been reimbursed at 85 % of Medicare allowable. Our practice had seen the opportunity to obtain the additional 15 % and had organized our schedules to allow for our physicians and nurse practitioners to be at the facility together. So, what the government was seeing was that I and my two nurse practitioners were each seeing 15 patients a day!

What I found most interesting was that when our attorney contacted the OIG investigators, it became apparent that they had no clue about what "incident-to" billing was. They were quickly educated, and phase two of our investigation came to a close. This wasn't the end of our "relationship" with the OIG. They had actually passed the investigation on to the state attorney general's office, and what I soon learned was that whenever a high-profile case was settled in our state, we would receive another subpoena for more billing records. We had become work for the state attorney general's office when they had nothing else to do! This process actually went on for the next few years. Every time that we received a subpoena, we would respond to it.

From the moment that we founded Senior Care of Colorado, we were extremely careful to educate all of our clinicians on proper coding and billing. We knew that this was of the utmost importance. In many ways, the ongoing government investigation forced us to maintain a process and discipline that would serve us very well in the coming years. In fact, one of the main concerns about the ongoing investigation was that our clinicians would start undercoding. We monitored this closely and maintained a lot of vigilance in assuring that our clinicians were trained in proper coding techniques. There were actually a couple of points along the way where we forgot to maintain our vigilance and appropriate coding dropped. This led to a decline in revenue. A geriatric practice cannot sustain undercoding for very long.

9.5   Trust Your Preparation

The last time that we received a government subpoena, I realized that they had decided to focus on a particular type of patient, many of whom were actually mine. These were patients that we saw frequently in our outpatient clinic. Once again, they were looking for patterns of abuse, but what they actually saw were patterns of excellent geriatric care. One patient whose chart was subpoenaed was a very dear patient of mine. He had severe congestive heart failure (CHF) and I actually saw him every 2 weeks in my office. This went on for almost 4 years, during which time he was never hospitalized! This is almost unheard of in a patient with his degree of CHF. I was actually saving a lot of money for Medicare, for the very low cost of frequent outpatient visits. When I saw that the government was reviewing this type of patient, I actually laughed, knowing that they wouldn't find any wrongdoing. At the same time, it was disturbing to me how much energy they continued to put in trying to find something. By this time, the investigation was not costing us any legal dollars, as our attorneys had told us that we knew what we were doing and didn't need to spend money on them.

How did our "relationship" with the government investigators end? This is both instructional and entertaining, although I didn't think so at the time. We received a call from a disabled homebound Medicare patient who lived in a rural area. He was diabetic and had a foot ulcer. Our nurse practitioner was doing house calls on him every week. We had identified certain types of patients who benefitted from weekly house calls. We believed strongly that this not only improved their care, but kept them out of the hospital. Well, this poor patient called us frantically, letting us know that a government investigator had come to interview him. I was so angry! It was one thing for the government to harass us, but to involve one of our frail homebound patients was another thing. I called our attorney and suggested that we make a big deal over this. He calmed me down and reminded me to let the sleeping dog lie. At the same time, he contacted the supervisor of the agent who interviewed our poor patient. I think the government finally realized the futility of their investigation. We never heard from them again.

What are the lessons in this? First of all, as I read everything I've written, I might be discouraged from ever practicing geriatrics. However, that really isn't the lesson. *The lesson is that it's important to understand and meticulously follow the coding and billing rules.* We were the largest practice of our kind in the country, so we became a target, and that was the cost of doing business for us. I hope that the government continues to refine its methods for identifying those who truly defraud the Medicare program, while not discouraging the rest of us who are trying to deliver good care to a population that desperately needs our attention. In the meantime, the reader should take note that despite a thorough and ongoing investigation of our practice, the government never found any wrongdoing.

Nursing Homes: Survival of the Fittest

10

When I came out of my geriatrics fellowship over 25 years ago, I had little interest in caring for people in nursing homes. Despite being a geriatrician and caring deeply about frail older adults, this setting was not appealing to me. Little did I know that 20 years later, nursing home care would be the primary reason that I was in a position to retire.

It is important to make it a priority to understand every other business that you interact with. Nursing homes are not only no exception but are a great example of why this rule is so important. The nursing home industry is one of the most complex arenas that you will ever work in. It is not surprising that in the 1990s, almost all of the publicly traded nursing home companies declared bankruptcy. This is one tough business to be successful in! Today, things haven't changed a lot in this regards, despite, or perhaps because of, the huge pressure to improve the quality of care that is delivered in nursing facilities.

One of the biggest things that has changed in the past 20 years is the type of care that is being delivered in nursing facilities. Twenty years ago it was common to stay in the hospital until you were "better," and then you went home. Today, the norm tends to be spending the required 3 days in the hospital before being sent out to a skilled nursing home for the remainder of your care. There has even been some shift in the treatment of certain illnesses that bypass the hospital and allow treatment directly in a nursing facility. Ironically, with both GeriMed and Senior Care of Colorado, we pioneered this approach in the managed care arena. There is every reason to believe that the chance to utilize nursing homes in this way will be even greater in the future. Because of this, there are numerous strategic opportunities that are certain to present themselves to geriatric practices. Positioning oneself to take advantage of these ever-changing circumstances will be a critical success factor.

10.1 Today's Nursing Homes

Let's take a look at the state of nursing homes today. Primarily in response to the reasons mentioned already, there has actually been a drive in the industry to create facilities that solely provide skilled nursing care post-hospitalization. These

© Springer International Publishing Switzerland 2016
M. Wasserman, *The Business of Geriatrics*, DOI 10.1007/978-3-319-28546-7_10

facilities do not provide long-term care. The reason for this is simple: money. Nursing facilities receive higher reimbursement if they provide skilled care. It has become a huge challenge to determine how to maximize this reimbursement in ways that allows facilities to deliver the necessary care while achieving profitability. Historically, nursing facilities that provided primarily long-term care services saw skilled care as a means of bolstering their bottom line. As freestanding "subacute" care facilities have popped up, this has provided negative pressure to more traditional facilities in their ability to provide a similar service.

Are skilled nursing facilities more profitable than long-term care facilities? From a pure economic perspective, there is greater revenue coming into a skilled facility, but their costs are appreciably greater due to increased nurse staffing needs and rehabilitative therapies. Not surprisingly, it is a chess match between the government, the insurers, and the facilities, trying to determine the appropriate cost of these services. The government wants to limit their expenditures and the facilities want to assure their profitability. In the old "cost-based" scenario, the government reimburses the facility for each day a patient is in a bed. This is similar to how hospitals were paid prior to the implementation of the DRG system. There is no question that the government is headed in the same direction with skilled nursing facilities. This is going to occur in many different ways. In an accountable care organization structure, it is actually possible that the ACO itself will be responsible for paying the facility. In a more traditional fee-for-service arrangement, the government is toying with bundled payments to the hospital for the entire length of care. Somehow, this payment will need to cover both the acute hospital and skilled nursing. It is also possible that there will be some type of DRG methodology put into play for skilled nursing facilities as well. The key is that providers must pay attention to which direction this goes. The approach that the geriatric clinician takes needs to take into account the prevailing payment methodologies in their local area.

Historically, the most costly part of the Medicare program has been acute hospital care. This typically accounts for over 33 % of all Medicare expenditures. Skilled nursing accounts for approximately 8 %. Hospitals are a huge lobby and absolutely do not want to have their share of Medicare expenditures reduced. The skilled nursing facility industry is far more fragmented and at a huge financial disadvantage. They also tend to be at the mercy of the hospitals when it comes to getting patients. In fact, nursing facilities have been trying forever to figure out how to get patients in their doors. With the advent of the readmission penalty, hospitals are now taking a far more critical look at where they send patients after discharge.

10.2 Patient Opportunities

With all of the above background come opportunities for geriatric healthcare providers. I am going to break this down into two areas. First is the skilled patient. Next is the long-term care patient. They are both important. In fact, I believe that one of the biggest mistakes a practice can make is to just choose one type of nursing home patient to follow. *The facility needs medical care provided to all of their patients and the practice needs to develop the most efficient workflow possible in any given building.*

It is important to realize that today's skilled nursing patient was yesterday's hospital patient. This provides a singularly unique opportunity for clinicians caring for patients in nursing homes. As one of the key elements of fee-for-service coding is the concept of "medical necessity," it actually isn't difficult to see the necessity of regularly seeing patients who historically were seen daily in the hospital setting in the not-too-distant past. Combined with the complexity and frailty of this population, regular visits make a lot of sense. Ironically, when viewed from a bundled or capitated payment perspective, regular visits can also make sense, with the caveat that the bundled rate must either cover the cost of provider visits or allow for shared savings in the reduction of overall costs. The approach to care in nursing facilities cannot be taken lightly. *The single most important clinical fact is that a frail older person in a nursing facility can decline rapidly in 24 h, and the only way to truly provide excellent care is with regular monitoring of the patient.*

It shouldn't be lost that the concept of coordinated care is a constant theme in the delivery of geriatric care. In the office setting, the practice will utilize its own staff. In the nursing home, it is an entirely different situation. In fact, many practices have gotten bogged down by trying to develop their own internal systems that interact with the nursing home system. This often leads to messages upon messages and lack of clarity of where medical decision-making is taking place. From a fee-for-service perspective, care delivered by the practitioner over the telephone, either personally or through a surrogate, is not billable. This becomes a pure cost center. The potential risk in the environment of alternative payment methods is that such systems will be seen as ways of saving provider time and money in the short term. There is also a move afoot to allow telehealth to be reimbursed in nursing facilities. This will definitely allow for revenue production, but will still require expenditures. As such, these systems may very well remain as cost centers. Additionally, critical analysis of the actual benefit to the patient has not been determined. Similarly, the impact on the overall cost of care of such programs is uncertain.

10.3   Interacting with the Nursing Facility

What many of these systems do is to add a third layer to the care of the nursing home resident. One has to wonder as to the overall value that this extra layer provides. The first layer is the actual nursing home staff who care for the resident on a daily basis. They see and hear what is going on with the individual resident. The second layer is the healthcare provider, in the form of the physician or perhaps their nurse practitioner or physician assistant. It should be easy to see how the ideal scenario is to have direct communication between these two layers. *Adding a third layer in the form of another nurse sitting at a computer with a headset brings multiple potential challenges.* Ideally, utilizing evidence-based protocols, that nurse can respond to the nursing home nurse with some type of order. It doesn't take a long time thinking about this process to realize that it would be simpler to educate the nursing facility nurses directly with such protocols and cut out the additional layer. The other problem is that frail elderly nursing home residents are individuals and don't always respond well to protocols that were written with the "average" patient in mind.

While it is often impossible for the nurse at the nursing facility to access the clinician immediately, the ultimate role of a triage system is to connect the clinician with the nurse in a timely fashion. There are also opportunities utilizing new technologies to achieve this goal. Over the years, I have seen failed systems where clinicians are overwhelmed with communications from nursing facilities. This issue takes on gargantuan proportions in the evening and overnight and is often a huge morale issue for practices. I have also seen incredibly robust systems that are prohibitively expensive, while not necessarily demonstrating evidence-based efficacy.

10.4   The Bottom Line

Here's the bottom line. In a fee-for-service environment, it is critical that a clinician lay eyes on the patient on a regular basis. This is good for care and good for reimbursement. It also lessens the amount of uncompensated time that is spent by both the facility nurses and the practice in trying to communicate. In an alternative payment environment, the only difference is in how the clinician assesses the patient. If new technologies allow for remote monitoring, it may not be as necessary for the clinician to be on site to assess the patient. Unfortunately, this is all new, and we really don't have adequate evidence one way or the other. In the meantime, *it still probably makes the most sense to enhance the availability of the clinician to assess the patient.*

How does a geriatric practice enhance the availability of a clinician to assess patients? Since there is presently a shortage of geriatricians, this becomes a key role for nurse practitioners and physician assistants. Clearly, they must be adequately trained in evaluating frail older adults. They must also be readily available. Some of our most successful nursing home practices involved having 1–2 FTEs in a building 5–7 days a week. It isn't hard to see a situation where one clinician comes to the facility between 6 and 7 a.m. and the other clinician doesn't leave the building until 7–8 p.m. These are actually ideal situations, as it allows for the clinicians to interact with both staff from all shifts and families at key times of the day.

While such comprehensive coverage is not always possible, it is actually not difficult to see how a practice dedicated to both caring for patients and developing excellent relationships with a nursing facility can achieve this type of coverage. *Comprehensive, "boots on the ground," provider coverage enhances communication with the facility and minimizes the need for phone calls and messages.* This level of collaboration also opens up the possibilities of educating nursing staff in the use of the practice's protocols, if they exist.

10.5   Medical Necessity

From the perspective of a fee-for-service-based practice, it is very easy to see the benefits of this type of practice model. Combined with the knowledge of time-based coding criteria, clinicians are in a position to provide the best care while on-site. I've often gotten pushback on this concept from those who question whether frequent visits will hold up under an intense audit. Here is the bottom line. *If a nurse, patient, or family member requests that the clinician see the patient, one has already established medical necessity. You can't say no!* If the clinician documents the reason they were asked to see the patient, they have given further documentation of medical necessity. If the clinician sees a patient 1 day, makes medication changes, and decides to look at the patient the very next day, that is good care. These are frail older adults who can undergo a rapid decline in just 24 h. *One just has to explain the reason for the visit to be paid under a fee-for-service arrangement.* It is also clear why this method works in a fee-for-service environment. The practice brings in revenue! The practice also minimizes costly off-site communication services that are of unproven value.

What about alternative payment methodologies? If the practice receives a lump sum for the care of the patient, frequent visits can appear to be costly. However, most alternative payment approaches will be tied to both utilization and quality targets. Hence, reducing unnecessary hospitalizations, procedures, and tests will save a lot of money. Improving quality measures will also be a benefit for both the practice and the nursing facility. Clearly, understanding the structure of the payment method is critical. For a practice to negotiate a set capitated rate without tying it to overall expenditures could easily turn out to be foolhardy. Ironically, an enlightened health plan will willingly pay for fee-for-service-based daily visits, all the while knowing that the cost of a single hospitalization will easily exceed the cost of those visits. The marketplace has long been aware of this, with the EverCare™ model being a prime example of this approach.

What about the nursing home itself? This is actually the most problematic aspect for a geriatric practice. I have described a practice model that *should* encourage a nursing facility to want to work with a practice. Yet, this doesn't always happen. Over the years I have seen many nursing homes make illogical decisions that they felt would increase their admissions. The stories are too numerous to share and many don't make sense, so I will not regale the reader with them. What is important, however, is how a practice needs to approach a facility in order to protect its own business interests. Once again, the ironic twist that shouldn't be surprising is that the focus needs to be on how to provide the best care and services for the patients.

10.6   Building Relationships

It is always critical for a practice to develop a relationship with both the administrator and the director of nursing. However, this relationship does not guarantee success, as maintaining excellent relations with the nursing staff is just as important. *Little things like thanking the staff for the work that they do is essential.* Similarly, responding to questions without acting like it is a burden is also important. How a practice responds to phone calls is also of great importance. If calls are not returned in a timely fashion, this will certainly lead to negative feedback. If your practice is in the facility on a daily basis, a call log can be very useful, so long as the clinicians make sure that they look at the log everyday. When used effectively, this method can be very beneficial to both the facility and the practice, saving a lot of time for both.

The interactions with the administrator and director of nursing take on other forms. The focus here needs to be on what the practice can do to help make the facility better. Are the providers well educated in the appropriate use of antipsychotic medications? Do they take a close look at admission medications from the hospital and discontinue inappropriate medications that might also be of high cost to the facility? Many clinicians are unaware that the facility is responsible for the cost of medications in skilled patients. Demonstrating this awareness to the administrator and director of nursing shows a level of partnership that will be perceived in a positive fashion.

10.7   Focus on Quality

Never discuss exchanging admissions to the facility in return for getting more patients! These are the types of discussions that can only put a practice in harm's way. The appropriate discussion has to do with how your practice will improve the quality of care provided by the facility. You should focus on how daily visits will reduce hospital readmission rates and help the facility with better quality indicators. Let the administrator know that the approach the practice takes to caring for their residents will also improve family and resident satisfaction. Most of us did not learn marketing skills in medical school, but *when it comes to delivering care in nursing facilities, those who ignore the customer will ultimately be at risk for losing business.*

Another facet of the relationship between a geriatric practice and nursing homes is that of being a medical director for the facility. Skilled nursing facilities are required by law to have medical directors. There are no specific requirements as to the skills and capabilities of that person, although I am hopeful that will change in the future. In the meantime, facilities will approach particular physicians for any number of reasons. One, they might think that they are finding a referral source. As I have mentioned previously, this is one discussion that is completely off-limits! Another reason a facility approaches you is that they recognize that you might have expertise in the area. Finally, and it is truly a shame that I must write this, the most common reason for choosing a medical director is that the facility needs a warm body to sign certain forms and policies. This should not be surprising in a healthcare environment that is still struggling to understand what geriatric medicine is all about.

It is not uncommon for geriatric practices to provider medical director services for some of the nursing facilities they serve clinically. It is actually a good idea, from the perspective of conflict of interest, to utilize a different clinician in the medical director role than the one caring for patients in the facility. However, in smaller communities, this may be impossible. In fact, there are circumstances where the medical director also acts as the attending physician for most, if not all, of the patients. We actually had a situation like this in a facility in rural Colorado where we sent clinicians weekly to provide care when no one else was available in the community to do so. Priorities become obvious in these types of situations.

I will leave the discussion of medical direction with an interesting story. Our practice had a relationship with a large nursing home chain. Not only did we provide care for many of the patients in their facilities, but we provided medical direction for all of their facilities. One day, I received a phone call that they were discontinuing all of our medical director contracts. Why? They had decided to offer their medical directorships to a hospitalist practice. The reasons for this decision should be obvious to the reader. The irony of this circumstance was that 6 months later an analysis of our operations in these buildings demonstrated an increase in patients, visits, and revenue! It is possible that having a clinician act as both an attending and medical director might actually detract from their focus on either of these roles.

There are still many communities around the country where nursing facilities have trouble finding clinicians who will come into their building to see patients. In these communities, a physician can build a significant practice just by walking in the door. One might ask why it is necessary to pay attention to how the practice treats the staff and interacts with the leadership when there is no competition. The answer is twofold. First, it's just good business. Second, you should develop a habit of hating surprises. Just because all of the existing business in a facility is handed to you on a platter today doesn't mean that will always be the case. It is also hard to break poor habits of individual clinicians. *Educating and encouraging physicians, nurse practitioners, and physician assistants on how to effectively interact with a nursing facility is a long-range investment that will pay off for many years to come.*

Assisted Living: Healthcare or Real Estate?

When we first opened the doors of Senior Care of Colorado, the idea of caring for residents in assisted living facilities wasn't even on our radar. However, it quickly became clear to us that a portion of our patient population resided in these facilities. They often had difficulty finding transportation to our offices. It struck us that there might be an opportunity for us to bring the care to them. There were a handful of other practices around the country that had started focusing on house calls and assisted living facilities. The problem was the reimbursement. At the time we started Senior Care, assisted living facilities were considered to be "domiciliary" facilities, and the Medicare reimbursement for seeing patients in such facilities was quite poor.

Despite the poor reimbursement, we decided to start sending our providers out to the assisted living facilities. No one else in Denver was doing this at the time, and everyone loved that we offered this new service. It wasn't difficult to grow our patient population. In the long run, this paid off in many ways for us. I'd like to say that we were brilliantly visionary, but we were probably just lucky. One thing we knew for sure is that the people who lived in assisted living facilities were the type of patients that we as geriatricians were trained to care for. They had multiple chronic illnesses and many had some degree of cognitive impairment.

11.1 Taking a Chance

Initially, our foray into assisted living facilities did not pay off financially. However, it was a relatively small part of our practice and definitely increased our favorability with home health agencies and nursing homes. A few years into our practice, through the extraordinary efforts of AMDA (American Medical Directors Association) and AAHCP (American Academy of Home Care Physicians), there was a significant increase in the reimbursement made for visits both in assisted living facilities and in patient's homes. While it would be interesting to hear an

© Springer International Publishing Switzerland 2016 79
M. Wasserman, *The Business of Geriatrics*, DOI 10.1007/978-3-319-28546-7_11

accounting of the politics of this achievement, most likely the RUC (the AMA's physician payment advisory committee) just didn't think that the overall impact of such visits would amount to much in the grander scheme of physician payment. For the most part, that has been true. On the other hand, we found ourselves in the right place at the right time. This is actually an important theme for geriatric practices. With the rapidly growing demographic of older adults, it is important to be cognizant of "where the action" is taking place. Being in the middle of it, regardless of reimbursement, leads to opportunities that create potential for both growth and success.

Assisted living facilities are another complex and often changing realm in the elder care continuum. For the most part, the industry has primarily been a "real estate play." The assets of the real estate become the key motivator for investors. Many of the large assisted living companies historically have outsourced the management of their facilities to outside management companies. One of the challenges of this dichotomy is that the "sweet spot" for these management companies has often been lacking. It has been fairly commonplace to find a lot of churning of the management companies, while the long-term goal on the real estate side is to hang tough through any real estate downturns.

11.2   The Decline of the Medical Model

When we started going to assisted living facilities, many of them had wellness nurses and were really trying to develop a business model that catered to their resident's medical issues. Over time, a lot of these programs fell by the wayside and we found facilities depending more and more on our services. This had the unique effect of further bolstering our care model. At the same time, it added additional stress to our providers who had to navigate these facilities without much assistance.

The assisted living facility industry has continued to struggle with this question. On one hand, by providing services that cater to addressing the health needs of their residents, they might prove more marketable. On the other hand, dealing effectively with the complex medical needs of the frail elderly provides plenty of opportunities for dissatisfied customers. There are additional challenges as a clinician when it comes to making recommendations to families in regard to such facilities when there is uncertainty as to the degree to which the facility focuses on the health and wellness of their residents.

On a positive note, we successfully navigated all of these changes in the industry, primarily by being aware of them. When facilities provided wellness nurses, we worked with them to coordinate the care of our patients and their residents. This was a win-win situation for both our practice and the facilities. When they didn't have a robust health and wellness program, we jumped in and were able to frequent the facility more often, satisfying the concerns of both patients and families.

While we have discussed the critical importance of nursing facilities in relation to the success of a geriatrics practice, assisted living facilities may soon be of equal, if not greater, importance. The healthcare landscape is changing, as is the continuum of care itself. There has been, and will continue to be, a move toward identifying the lowest cost setting for the frail elderly to be cared for. We have already moved from the "old days," where an older adult spent 4–6 weeks in the hospital, to a 3-day hospital stay followed by a 2–3-week nursing facility stay. It doesn't take a lot of foresight to envision the utilization of assisted living facilities as yet another lower-cost environment around which to allow older adults to convalesce and undergo rehabilitation.

11.3 Choosing the Most Appropriate Level of Care

The critical balance that must be considered in determining the most appropriate level of care for a frail older adult is that of the necessary nursing, or skilled, services that are required. As a geriatrician, it has always been clear that the most important facet in the successful care of the elderly patient is the nostrum of *do not harm*. Procedures, tests, and medications are all fraught with the possibility of adverse reactions. Often, what the patient needs the most is a caring hand. Attention to good nutrition and maintaining function through activity can be the most important factor in the recovery of an older adult from an acute illness. In many ways, this doesn't require highly skilled caregivers, with a few key exceptions. The skills that they need are not medical, but interpersonal. This is where a high-quality assisted living experience can actually be more helpful than the hospital or nursing home. But there is a fine balance. Bringing medical care into the facility can help to assure this balance.

Delivering primary care services in an assisted living facility requires a certain level of sophistication. Every facility is set up differently. There are a multitude of key elements that must be mastered. Who is responsible for giving the resident their medications? What is the process for this to occur? How and when does the resident eat? What is their diet like? If there is the need for additional caregiver support, what are the costs? Is there an outside home health agency? Some facilities now will have their own agency. What is the level of home health care that is being provided? How engaged is the family?

11.4 Planning Matters

We found it very useful to schedule regular provider time in assisted living facilities. It is important that there be a degree of certainty and continuity available for both residents and staff. It is also critical to coordinate with the patient's family prior to a visit. The last thing you want to do is to see the patient and be unable to contact their daughter at the same time. Not connecting with the family at the time of the visit can lead to a long, uncompensated, phone call later in the day. The practice needs to invest in someone who is arranging for the visit to be coordinated with the family. The concept of the clinician bringing a "scribe" along is relatively new and works very well in the assisted living environment. This person can make sure that the patient is ready and can also coordinate with family and caregivers to assure timely and effective communication. This can even help with documentation while the clinician is seeing the patient. The cost of such a person pales in comparison to the value of the time of the clinician and needs to be balanced with the impact of positive efficiencies.

The opportunity to coordinate care and to fully involve the patient and family in the care plan is one of the greatest potential advantages of delivering care in an assisted living facility. This type of care doesn't occur on its own and definitely takes planning, process, and structure. To say that most assisted living facilities appreciate this would be an understatement. The process begins with understanding how the facility works. If there is a wellness nurse on site, it is critical to develop a relationship with this person. They must be given the utmost respect, and it is critical to assure that one's practice does not operate at odds with the wellness nurse. The nurse will be grateful to a practice that reaches out and seeks to collaborate. Some wellness nurses will maintain a chart for the resident. This is a certainty if the facility provides any degree of medication management. It is often useful to keep a copy of one's note in such a chart, although this should not be assumed to be the patient's medical record. This is different from the medical record in a nursing facility, where it is certainly appropriate to maintain that record as the sole repository for clinician's notes.

11.5   The Challenge of Wellness Nurses

Wellness nurses will have a great degree of variation in skill set and abilities. While some will only be proficient in checking temperature and blood pressure, others may have the ability to evaluate and report on a resident's condition. How a practice responds to this is dependent on the skill level of the caregiver in the facility. Assisted living facilities are not regulated to the degree of skilled nursing homes, which places an added burden on the clinician to recognize the validity of any clinical information that they receive. It is thus very important for the practice to inconspicuously assess the skills of a wellness nurse. As the person in these positions may change frequently, this becomes an ongoing process.

The skills of a wellness nurse are not the only important aspect to pay attention to. This person will have their own philosophy regarding the medical needs of the residents. We have found most wellness nurses to be relatively holistic and to not desire that their residents are on a lot of medications. However, that is not always the case. On occasion, a wellness nurse may have been indoctrinated into a more traditional approach to the medical care of older individuals and may try to encourage the use of medications. This can be a very tricky situation, as the practice needs to balance the needs of the resident with the cooperation of the wellness nurse. It is easy to see that if the practice's providers clash with the wellness nurse, a collaborative environment would be lacking.

11.6   Creating a Bridge

Clinician's caring for their patients in an assisted living facility must create a bridge between the patient, family, and staff. They must take great pains not to get in the middle of disputes between the patient and the facility. The primary reason for this is just the simple fact that effective communication is critical in order to deliver appropriate geriatric medical care. There is a broader reason that the average clinician generally does not pay attention to. There is a marketing role that is necessary in order to develop and maintain a good relationship with an assisted living facility. Physicians, nurse practitioners, and physician assistants have not been taught marketing during their training. Marketing is not only important to assure a steady flow of patients, but it is also very important in developing relationships that support effective communication. The days of a physician being gruff with staff in an assisted living facility or nursing home are gone. Not only the care of the patient, but the business itself can suffer from such behavior.

With the advent of chronic care management codes, there may be an opportunity in the future to utilize these codes for a more coordinated approach to caring for residents of assisted living facilities. In the meantime, time-based coding still provides a highly effective method for doing everything that is necessary for the care of the patient. Cell phones make it very easy to communicate with the patient's family during the visit. Furthermore, if there is any need to involve or interact with a specialist, the time to make that call and communicate it with the patient is during the face-to-face visit itself. The clinician's note should be written while in the company of the patient for multiple reasons. The first reason, as always, is to assure that the impression and plan are directly communicated to the patient and hopefully to the key family member at the time of the visit. *There is nothing worse than telling mom that you are adjusting her medication and then getting an angry phone call from her daughter later in the day.*

As noted earlier in this chapter, it may be worthwhile to bring a medical assistant along to the facility, especially if there are a large number of patients to be seen. Patients have a remarkable ability to disappear in even the smallest facility, and having someone who can make sure that the next patient is ready to be seen can save precious minutes with each patient. A medical assistant can also prepare the necessary information, such as reviewing a medication list and even checking the medication cabinet for both prescription and nonprescription drugs. This works especially well if the clinician is billing using the traditional E&M criteria but still saves time under any circumstance.

11.7   Clinician Availability

Having clinicians available for urgent visits is also a critical factor in the ongoing success of a geriatric practice that visits assisted living facilities. The key to making this work is to focus on geography when it comes to looking at how the clinicians spend their time. Pairing specific assisted living facilities with local nursing homes allows for a clinician to break away from routine visits in a nursing facility and urgently visit a patient in a nearby assisted living facility.

Today, with the growth of pure house call practices, there has been an appropriate move into assisted living facilities by such practices. One of the problems that they run into is not having the hub of a clinic-based practice, although advancing technology may help with this. The other problem with pure house call practices is the limited ability to provide urgent visits, especially when the practice is relatively small. This is the main reason that we have historically picked up patients from house call practices that were unable to provide the type of availability that facilities will appreciate from a robust geriatric practice.

11.8   Finding the Sweet Spot

There are a multitude of reasons for a geriatric practice to consider providing care in assisted living facilities. The "sweet spot" for high-cost patients (from the insurers' perspective) resides in these facilities. The structure of an assisted living facility is such that it provides an excellent locale for the delivery of direct medical care to their residents. From a public relations perspective, families are enthralled that they don't have to take mom or dad to the doctor's office. Facilities appreciate not having to provide transportation as well, a fact that has been made abundantly clear during times of high gasoline prices. Geriatricians are in the right time, and assisted living facilities definitely appear to be one of the right places!

House Calls: A "New" Old-Fashioned Approach

12.1 House Calls from a Bygone Era

A few years ago, I had the opportunity to visit New England during the fall colors. We ran across a rural ranch in Vermont where a "gentleman" doctor had lived until the early 1990s. He passed away in his 90s having been in telephone contact with an ill patient the same day he died. It turns out that this doctor had been doing house calls for over 60 years. His original nurse had passed away, only to be replaced by her niece, in the doctor's office that existed on his property. There was a horse and buggy that he had used for house calls many years earlier. It turns out that back in the horse and buggy days, physicians had special horses that they used at night. The horses knew their way back home, so that the doctor could get some necessary sleep! I remember wishing that I had known about this doctor while he was still alive. I would have loved to have met him. It certainly seemed to me that they don't make doctors like that anymore.

Physicians have done house calls since the beginning of time. Unfortunately, the advent of Medicare probably impacted the ability of doctors to perform house calls more than one would like to admit. The reasons, simply stated, are the rules and the reimbursement. Over the past 50 years, house calls have become a very rare occurrence, performed only by the most dedicated clinicians. In fact, they have literally been relegated to fond memories of a time past. The last television doctor who did house calls was Marcus Welby, not surprisingly in the 1960s. Today, there is beginning to be a resurgence of the house call concept. It has happened for many reasons, yet it is not as simple of a delivery model as it would seem. For this reason, I will focus on the various angles around which one should plan a home visit program.

When we opened Senior Care of Colorado in 2001, we were very cautious with the use of house calls. We realized that, as geriatricians, there ought to be a place for home visits. We also realized that we needed to be profitable, and how we structured a house call program would be critical to its long-term success. Before I go into the logistics of a successful house call practice, it is worthwhile to review the reasons for and the value of home visits.

© Springer International Publishing Switzerland 2016
M. Wasserman, *The Business of Geriatrics*, DOI 10.1007/978-3-319-28546-7_12

12.2   The Stress of the Office Visit

It has always been remarkable to me to see how a patient looks in my office versus how they look sitting in a hospital bed. The milieu that we observe our patients in influences our perceptions of how the patient is doing. As a geriatrician, I was trained to do home visits. One of the first things I learned was how much more comfortable patients looked in their own home. The concept of "white coat hypertension" quickly comes to mind when thinking about how the setting that we see patients in might influence their objective physical findings. Going to a doctor's appointment is fraught with numerous complexities that can affect how a patient might present to us. First of all, as noted, is their blood pressure. There is every reason to believe that their blood pressure might be elevated just from the stress of knowing that they are visiting the doctor. What other physical findings might be similarly impacted?

There are many other factors that impact how a patient looks when they finally arrive in the exam room. If the patient has any degree of frailty, the exertion necessary to get dressed, travel, and then walk into our office is enough to tire them out. Then, they have to wait in the waiting area for up to an hour if we are behind schedule. I suppose that if we're trying to find things wrong, having a patient come in for an appointment will improve the likelihood of that happening!

Patients, and family members for that matter, who see us in the office are often like deers in the headlights. The doctor appointment experience can be overwhelming and they will often forget a lot of what is discussed. They might also forget to tell us some of the key reasons that they were even there for a visit! If the patient has any degree of cognitive impairment, these issues are heightened by the unfamiliar surroundings of the physician's office.

Most medical offices are not built with the frail older patient in mind. There may not be handrails in the hallway. The exam rooms might be cramped. The staff may rush the patient into the room. Exam tables are generally not friendly to a frail older adult. Parking may be difficult and there may be a significant walk to the office itself.

12.3   The Value of House Calls

When we see our patients in their own homes, the dynamics changes completely. First of all, they aren't waiting for us in an unfamiliar place with nothing to do. In fact, if we are running behind, they can go about their routine daily tasks. They don't have to travel to our office; they can be seen in the comfort of their own home, preferably sitting on their favorite chair or sofa. This setup offers a huge opportunity to assure a positive interaction between the patient and the clinician. I can't begin to share the number of times I spent the first 5 min of an office visit listening to a patient or family member complain about their having had to wait an hour to be seen. Not only is the time spent not productive, but the interpersonal relationship between the doctor and patient gets off on the wrong foot.

Another important opportunity that home visits create is the ability to review a patient's medications, including their over-the-counter medications. This is fundamentally important on so many levels. First, we can see how they have their medications arranged and what system they are using to take them. Second, we will see if they are also taking additional supplements such as herbs or vitamins. We also have the opportunity to peek into their refrigerator and get an idea of potential nutritional issues that might be occurring. Finally, we can see the overall status of their living environment. I have seen a number of patients who are "pack rats," and it is hard to even navigate getting around their home. A visual review of the home allows us to look for fall risk factors.

It is also important to take the time while visiting the patient in their home to speak to family members who are concerned and have a stake in their health. It is invariably the daughter, but can also be the son who lives a thousand miles away. I remember a very unique and complex 95-year-old patient of mine who was on hemodialysis (yes, you read that correctly). Her son was a physician who lived far away. The daughter would actually come to the house for my home visits. Each time, we would call the son and answer his questions. The daughter would thank me profusely, because historically she had been the one that translated the content of a doctor's visit to her physician brother. It inevitably didn't work out well, until I started doing house calls on her mom.

12.4   Chronic Disease and the Value of Home Visits

I once had a patient who spent half of his year living in the island nation of Tonga. While he lived in Tonga, his health seemed to be fine. As soon as he came to Denver, his health would fall apart, with his diabetes getting out of control and his congestive heart failure acting up. Oftentimes, if we didn't see him shortly after his return to the United States, he would end up in the hospital. He would typically have several hospitalizations over the course of several months. Then he would return to Tonga, and the cycle would repeat itself. Finally, we set up a system where we would be alerted when he returned from his annual trip to Tonga. As soon as we knew that he was back in town, we would set up a home visit with one of our physician assistants. We continued to do house calls weekly while he was in town. The hospitalizations stopped!

My physician assistant came to me once and asked why we continued to do weekly house calls when everything seemed stable. My response was that it was working and that we often do more by just touching and observing complex chronically ill patients than by aggressively treating them. Due to a series of scheduling snafus, our team missed the patient's weekly house calls for a few weeks. He ended up in the hospital. While I would normally hesitate to state my case for a care approach with what appears to be anecdote, I have had many similar experiences. In fact, my standard approach to frail older adults with multiple hospital admissions has been regular home visits. Invariably, the hospitalizations grind to a halt.

12.5   Independence at Home

The American Academy of Home Care Physicians is a society made up of physicians who perform house calls. Many of them have had similar experiences as the one I shared above and believe that regular visits by a clinician to the home of a frail older adult can improve quality and reduce costs. The "Independence at Home Act" was passed with their urging and support and has put into place a demonstration project that aims to prove the effectiveness of delivering comprehensive primary care services at home in Medicare beneficiaries with multiple chronic conditions. The demonstration also rewards healthcare providers that provide high-quality care while reducing costs. The outcomes in the first year of the demonstration were positive. These are the type of opportunities that geriatricians have been waiting for! It is also potentially the tip of a very large iceberg. Interestingly, many of the practices involved in the demonstration are self-contained home visit practices, which make their results even more profound. I think it should not be lost that there are huge opportunities to scale this model and improve efficiencies utilizing the resources of a larger practice that manages care throughout the entire continuum.

12.6   Scaling a Home Visit Program

One of the great advantages that we had at Senior Care of Colorado was the fact that we ultimately had over 65 clinicians, many of whom were in the field on a daily basis. Under this scenario, it is possible to draw a geographic circle around a provider and the nursing homes and assisted living facilities where they provide care. Within this circle becomes the opportunity to provide timely home visits. One of the more interesting sidelights that we have observed are very successful solo home visit programs that outgrow themselves when the provider is challenged to be in two places at one time across town. In fact, we grew our home visit program when some of these very "successful" programs dissolved under the weight of such growth.

At the start of a solo physician house call practice, the clinician is able to be available daily and is also not constrained in the time he or she spends with the patient. As the practice grows, constraints begin to occur. The clinician can't spend as much time, and acute visits become much more difficult. The practice needs the working capital to hire an additional provider at that point in order to grow. Until the practice has several providers, this can prove to be a very challenging situation.

Economies of scale are very important in any business, and a house call operation is no exception. If a patient needs an urgent visit, telling them to go to the emergency room or urgent care defeats the purpose on multiple levels. Even a pure fee-for-service model will not work under these circumstances due to patient satisfaction issues. A shared savings model will definitely fail under the weight of increased costs if patients are forced to utilize the emergency room rather than receive a timely home visit. Telemedicine may bring some additional efficiencies to this model, albeit it may still be important to have a live clinician on-site. However, this might be a nurse or LPN if the physician, nurse practitioner, or physician assistant can't make it to the home.

It should be obvious to see how a geriatrics practice that focuses on nursing home and assisted living facilities is well positioned to develop a home visit program. Clinicians "in the field" are less constrained by a specific schedule. If they are within a short distance of a home visit patient who needs an acute visit, it is much easier to leave the nursing home than it would be to leave a busy office practice. Ironically, a pure house call practice doesn't really have anything for a clinician to do during any "downtime." The combination has the potential to be very powerful and can take advantage of economies of scale.

12.7   The House Call of the Future

As noted above, new technologies may bring all sorts of opportunities to the home visit arena. The ability to transmit audiovisual information, as well as other technical information, could easily change the way we deliver home visits. I admit that I am somewhat old fashioned in this regard and still cling to the idea of observing, touching, and feeling my patients in person. With that said, having a less expensive clinician on-site and utilizing technology to pass on information are certainly possibilities. Furthermore, as technology improves it is certainly possible that the interface we have will provide an "in-person" feel to the experience. Other potential technologic advances include the ability to do on-site testing such as a cbc or electrolyte panel in real time. Ultrasonic and other noninvasive testing is also possible. There is no question that being able to accomplish all of this in the comfort of a patient's own home is very appealing.

The ability to bring necessary treatments to patients in their own home has certainly expanded over the past couple of decades. Intravenous therapies and other modalities are certainly possible and enhance the potential for managing patients without an acute hospitalization. The psychological factor of staying in one's home cannot be discounted, although further research could certainly add to our knowledge base.

12.8   The Business Case for House Calls

A robust home visit program that is part of a comprehensive geriatric practice can definitely be of value in a fee-for-service environment. Our experience at Senior Care of Colorado definitely demonstrated this. On the other hand, in the setting of alternate payment models such as shared savings arrangements or bundled payments, there appears to be a huge financial opportunity. There is one caveat. Actuarially, one must be cautious with a small number of patients in a risk or shared savings environment. A few very complex patients can wipe out any savings from all of your other patients. In this regard, a home visit program that is part of a much larger at-risk population of ambulatory patients certainly makes the most sense.

Home visits also present a significant marketing opportunity. What patient doesn't want to be part of a practice that provides house calls? Families are incredibly supportive as it reduces their involvement in assuring that mom gets to the doctor. There is actually literature and anecdotal experience that physicians who perform house calls are at less risk for malpractice suits. I hope that I will be proven wrong about the bygone era and the type of doctors available who are dedicated to doing whatever it takes for their patients.

Care Coordination

13

When I became a geriatric fellow in 1988, I got interested in some published research about the "channeling" studies. These were some of the first major prospective studies evaluating case management in the elderly population. The findings were less than impressive, which concerned me. As a geriatrician, I had assumed that case management would be helpful. What was the problem? The issue then, which I believe continues to this day, is that case management or care coordination that is not integrated into the primary care of a patient is often doomed to failure. There may be exceptions to this, but most of those exceptions will probably occur in programs where the care coordination process is actually able to impact medical decision making.

13.1 Care Coordination Rounds

When I joined Kaiser Permanente directly out of my fellowship, I began looking for ways to impact the care of older adults in the system. This ultimately led to the development of "care coordination rounds." I would round with the hospital's discharge planners every day. In doing this, I was able to identify many situations where the geriatric approach to care differed from the more traditional approach that was being taken. First, I would have the discharge planner pass on our suggestions to the physician. As one might imagine, this did not always work. I found myself contacting the patient's physician to make suggestions, some of which were followed. This was not an easy task for someone with my personality type. I have always disliked confrontation, and physicians generally don't take kindly to being told to do something differently.

13.2 The Importance of Physician to Physician Communication

One of the rules that I was to learn even more decisively a few years later was that the most effective way to communicate with a physician is to have another physician make that communication. I personally don't believe that this should be

© Springer International Publishing Switzerland 2016   91
M. Wasserman, *The Business of Geriatrics*, DOI 10.1007/978-3-319-28546-7_13

necessary, but on a practical level, it is definitely the most effective way to engage another doctor. Granted, even then, the physicians that I would contact would often respond negatively. I was the young geriatrician. What did I know? I certainly learned that coming across as a "know it all" was not the best approach. I would typically ask them if they had considered alternative approaches, and that in my experience, these might also work. Sometimes I would gently ask that they try a different approach. Some physicians were always resistant. Others went along with my suggestions to get me out of their hair. Human nature is certainly an interesting aspect to any approach we might take.

Over time, I do believe that the physicians that I worked with realized that my suggestions were not outlandish. Oftentimes, we would make suggestions that clearly improved the overall coordination of care. This would actually lead to a lower burden on the physician themselves. I began to discover new ways of phrasing my questions. One of my favorite approaches was to ask the doctor if they would hospitalize the patient that day if they were to see them in the office with their present set of circumstances. This was always the most intriguing approach. Many patients look lousy at the time of admission and the decision to hospitalize is easy. Three days later, they look much better, but the physician is waiting for a lab result, or trying to "fine-tune" their medications. This would always be the key focal point. *If they had actually walked into their office that day, looking better, but needing additional "fine-tuning," would they admit them to the hospital?*

13.3   Outpatient Geriatric Consultation

In addition to our care coordination rounds, which were clearly successful, we developed an outpatient geriatric consult clinic. The clinic was composed of myself, a nurse practitioner, a social worker, a geriatric pharmacist, and a geriatric nurse specialist who acted as our care coordinator. The biggest learning experience I had from this clinic was that not all physicians followed our recommendations, although in many cases, we became the de facto primary care physician for the patient. It was in those circumstances that the care coordination model worked the best!

The best examples of effective care coordination models include PACE (Program for All Inclusive Care of the Elderly) and GRACE (Geriatric Resources for Assessment and Care of Elders). There are other programs and models, but what most of them have in common are the geriatric approach to care and methods for effectively coordinating that care. In an earlier chapter, I shared how we put together our care coordination model in Orlando. It is important that a program fully understand the role of care coordination services. At GeriMed of America, we developed a fairly comprehensive outline of the role of care coordination services and guidelines which drove the workflow, which are both necessary for rolling out an effective care coordination model. I will share these below and believe that they provide an excellent starting point for any care coordination program.

13.3.1 Role of Care Coordination Services

Care coordination personnel are responsible for the coordination of care of the MedWise™ Center patient throughout the entire continuum of care. They assist the physician in developing and carrying out an appropriate plan of care, when applicable. They are an integral part of the interdisciplinary team and work to provide and ensure the delivery of appropriate and cost-effective quality care and services to all patients and their families. They assist in allowing the physician to provide the delivery of the Geriatric Medical Model of Care and help patients and caregivers in understanding this Model.

Care coordination personnel are responsible for ensuring that the following are carried out:

1. Psychosocial and general health screening of all patients entering the MedWise™ Center.
2. Further assessment for applicable MedWise™ Center patients.
3. The appropriate assessment level is determined for all MedWise™ Center patients.
4. Specific activities are carried out based upon each patient's assessment level.
5. A plan of care is developed as deemed applicable by the physician and the care coordination personnel.
6. Advance directives are discussed with and/or provided to each patient or authorized agent.
7. Necessary information is entered into the Care Management System.
8. MedWise™ Center patients and their families/caregivers are educated as to the Geriatric Medical Model of Care and the Geriatric Medical Approach to Practice.
9. The MedWise™ Center staff has appropriate knowledge of and relationships with pertinent agencies and community resources, allowing for the most effective care of the Center patients.
10. Situations of noncompliance with medications and treatment plan are assessed.
11. Family counseling and education are provided as needed in order to facilitate any transition through the continuum of care.
12. Appropriate discharge planning occurs from the emergency room, hospital, and subacute and home healthcare and is coordinated with the physician and the patient's family/caregivers.
13. Crisis intervention occurs, and protective agencies for the safety and protection of Center patients are notified when appropriate.
14. Weekly care coordination team meetings occur.
15. Programs/inservices/classes for the patient population occur on a regular basis.
16. The physician and interdisciplinary team identify the most appropriate, cost-effective level of care for each individual patient.

13.3.2 Guidelines for Care Coordination Services

1. Psychosocial and general health screening will be provided to all patients entering the MedWise™ Center.
   (a) Each patient will receive an information packet that includes an explanation of care coordinator services.
   (b) A Short Form Assessment and general health screening will be completed on or before the patient's first visit.
   (c) Standardized tests including, but not limited to, the Geriatric Depression Scale and the Folstein Mini-Mental State Exam will be administered based upon the physician's evaluation.
2. An appropriate assessment level is determined for all MedWise™ Center patients.
   (a) A "risk level" can be entered in the Care Management System (CMS) if appropriate following the first patient visit and the completion of the Short Form Assessment.
   (b) If the initial review indicates the need for a more in depth evaluation, this will occur within three office visits or 60 days.
   (c) An appropriate knowledge of the patient's financial resources.
   (d) All patients having evidence of potential for unsafe driving will be reported to the DMV, and they and their family will be advised of the recommendation not to drive any motor vehicle. Pertinent state law will be followed in regard to this issue.
   (e) All new patients are reviewed at the weekly care conference.
3. Specific activities are carried out based on each patient's assessment.
   (a) Each patient's risk level will determine the appropriate activities.
4. A plan of care is developed as deemed applicable by the physician and the care coordination personnel.
   (a) The plan of care will be based on information gathered from the initial assessment tools, discussion with the physician, and care conferences.
   (b) The patient will be allowed to participate in the development of the plan of care to the maximum degree possible.
   (c) The plan of care will be composed of pertinent clinical and nonclinical activities.
   (d) Care coordination personnel will be responsible for overseeing the delivery of the plan of care.
   (e) Care coordination personnel will be responsible for assuring that the plan of care is reevaluated as the patient's condition or risk level changes.
5. Advance directives are discussed with and/or provided to each patient or authorized agent.
   (a) Advance directives will be addressed within three office visits or 60 days from the first visit, whichever occurs first.
   (b) The patient will be provided with information relating to advance directives, and staff will be available to discuss this issue with patients. Patients declining to provide information regarding advance directives will be referred to their physician for further discussion.

(c) All advance directive information is entered in the Care Management System immediately.

6. Necessary information is entered into the Care Management System.
   (a) Necessary information includes, but is not limited to, all activities carried out by care coordination personnel.
   (b) All requests for support services.
   (c) Specific utilization information including acute hospital, skilled nursing, home care, DME, and specialty referrals.
   (d) Advance directive information.
   (e) Emergency party information.
   (f) Patient status changes, e.g., change from active to nursing home patient.

7. Educating MedWise™ Center patients and their families/caregivers as to the Geriatric Medical Model of Care.
   (a) Patient's and families are educated as to the Geriatric Medical Model and Approach to Care.
   (b) All patient's and family's questions regarding the approach to care are addressed.

8. The MedWise™ Center staff has appropriate knowledge of and relationships with pertinent agencies and community resources, allowing for the most effective care of the Center patients.
   (a) Information on agencies and community resources will be collected in order to ensure the ability to provide quality care to our patients.
   (b) An ongoing relationship with agencies and community resources will be maintained.
   (c) The value of each agency and resource will be continually evaluated and information kept up to date.

9. Situations of noncompliance with medications and treatment plan are assessed.
   (a) Patients will be assessed for possible interventions and alternatives, such as prepackaged medications or assistance at home.
   (b) Patients will be assessed for appropriate education and/or interventions in order to maximize compliance with the treatment plan.

10. Appropriate discharge planning occurs from the emergency room, hospital, and subacute and home healthcare and is coordinated with the physician and the patient's family/caregivers.
   (a) Once a physician has determined that a patient is appropriate for discharge, that discharge should occur that same day.
   (b) Family concerns about the discharge plan or process should be addressed.
   (c) Appropriate suggestions should be made by care coordination personnel to assist the physician in identifying the most appropriate, cost-effective level of care for each individual patient.
   (d) Follow-up visits should be established at the time of discharge.

11. Weekly care coordination team meetings will occur.
   (a) All new patients will be reviewed at this time.
   (b) All monitored, case managed, and crisis managed patients will be discussed at this time.

12. Care coordination personnel will have knowledge of all globally capitated managed care plans the MedWise™ Center participates in, as well as specific plan benefits.
13. Care coordination personnel will have knowledge of all ancillary and skilled nursing facility arrangements including both capitated and per diem available under any globally capitated arrangements.
14. Programs/inservices/classes for the patient population and general public will occur on a regular basis. Care coordination personnel will:
    (a) Be responsible for setting up regular educational programs for the MedWise™ patient population and the general public
    (b) Be responsible for assisting with the delivery of any Wellness and Exercise Programs
    (c) Participate in referral development activities for the MedWise™ Center

13.3.3   Risk Assessment Levels and Criteria

13.3.3.1 Independent
Indicator
Patients who are functionally independent and/or have adequate formal and informal support with no stated or assessed psychosocial needs

Activity
1. Patient-related contact as needed, with a minimum contact of one (1) telephone call every 6 months
2. Additional contact as requested by patient, family/caregiver, or other member of the interdisciplinary team

13.3.3.2 Monitored
Indicators (included but not necessarily limited to):
1. Patients who have limited formal and informal supports
2. The presence of caregiver/family stress or emotional problems
3. The presence of mental health concerns such as depression or anxiety
4. Patients with multiple health problems and/or functional disabilities
5. Patients with financial difficulties
6. Patients who were previously case managed but whose situation has stabilized
7. Patients who were previously independent but whose situation has declined
8. Patients who are being case managed by other agencies
9. Patients who reside in assisted living residencies, board, and care homes or group homes
10. Patients with poor cognitive functioning (memory loss, confusion, or poor judgment).

Activity (included but not necessarily limited to):
1. There will be patient related contact at each office visit.
2. There will be a telephone call to patient and/or family/caregiver every 1–3 months.

3. There will be a minimum of at least one quarterly review in care conference.
4. Discussion with community/private case managers, if any, once every quarter, preferably before clinic care conference.
5. Additional contact as requested by patient, family/caregiver, or other member of the MedWise Center team.

13.3.3.3 Case Managed
Indicators (included but not necessarily limited to):
1. Patients who require frequent and/or intense contact in order to maintain a level of functioning which will enable them to remain in the least restrictive environment possible at the time
2. Patients who were previously monitored but whose condition has declined
3. Patients with acute episodes or exacerbation's of the conditions listed as indicators for monitored
4. Patients with poor nutrition
5. Patients with multiple hospital admissions
6. Patients in more advanced stages of memory disorders and living at home or with caregivers (family or other)
7. Patients with significant loss and bereavement issues

Activity (included but not necessarily limited to):
1. There will be patent-related contact at each office visit.
2. There will be telephone contact with patient or family/caregiver every month.
3. Discussion with community involved case manager, if any, once every month.
4. Review in care conference once each month.
5. Additional contact as requested by patient, family/caregiver, or other member of the MedWise Center team.

13.3.3.4 Crisis Management
Indicator
Acute situation requiring immediate intervention on a short-term basis

13.4 The Value of Care Coordination

There are certainly practical issues surrounding the ultimate effectiveness of a care coordination model. As I recounted in the earlier chapter, one has to spend money to make money. Investing in care coordination is worthwhile if a practice benefits from the outcomes of having such a program. This clearly works in a practice or program where reducing overall healthcare costs brings in additional revenue. In a purely fee-for-service practice, the care coordination model has historically been lacking due to its cost without any return on the investment. The recent development of care coordination codes has opened the door to address this. It is likely that the format and reimbursement for these codes will continue to evolve, hopefully making them cost-effective for a geriatric practice. On the other hand, if a practice is part of an ACO or participates in a shared savings model, the decision to provide these services will ultimately be made simply by doing a cost/benefit analysis.

The experiences of GeriMed of America and Senior Care of Colorado can teach us one thing. A care coordination model integrated into a practice that is driven by a geriatric approach to care can certainly be profitable! As we have shown in other chapters, one must also have the financial acumen to assure that the revenue that stems from these types of programs is captured.

Medicare Advantage: Past, Present, and Future

14

For many of us who became physicians in the past 30 years, it may seem like managed care organizations have been around forever. Not only is that not the case, but the growth of this type of approach to healthcare has only occurred on a national basis in the fairly recent past. Like anything new, I think that it's important to realize that we might not have it all figured out at this point in time. Taking a look at where this approach began and what has become of it, particularly in the context of my practice experience over the past 30 years, is informative.

My curiosity about managed care began when I read about the Marshfield Clinic while I was a geriatric Fellow. In 1971, the first rural Health Maintenance Organization (HMO) was born in Marshfield, Wisconsin. It ultimately did not succeed for a variety of reasons. While prepaid health plans have been around since the early twentieth century, HMO's didn't really begin to grow until the HMO Act of 1973, which encouraged their development. By the time I started my residency in 1985, HMOs were expanding, and I happened to have one of the largest ones in the country in my backyard. Looking to make some extra money during my internal medicine residency, I began moonlighting at Kaiser-Permanente in Woodland Hills, California. I worked in the urgent care clinic in the evening and also worked in the hospital at night. This was my introduction to the world of HMOs.

14.1 Geriatrics and HMOs

While in the first year of my geriatric Fellowship, I was approached by the Chief of Internal Medicine at Kaiser, Woodland Hills. Did I want to start a geriatrics program? I had read the existing research about managed care. I was also very familiar with the research on care coordination at the time. It was clear to me that geriatrics was about an interdisciplinary approach. It was also clear to me that the geriatric approach to care seemed to be very cost-effective. As a geriatrician, I had been trained that hospitalization was to be avoided if possible. I also tried to minimize

© Springer International Publishing Switzerland 2016
M. Wasserman, *The Business of Geriatrics*, DOI 10.1007/978-3-319-28546-7_14

procedures and medications. It just made sense that the HMO approach was the ideal setting for geriatrics.

Timing is everything in life. Geriatrics was a young speciality in 1989. This looked like an excellent opportunity. There were not many geriatricians around at the time, which I think ultimately led to the difficulty that geriatrics had in gaining traction in the managed care world. With that said, I left my fellowship program after 1 year and jumped head first into the world of managed care.

14.2 Utilization Management

The number one focus of managed care in the 1990s was utilization management. Nurses were trained to look for excessive use of resources. Hospitals were doing this because of the DRG system and the desire to save money by discharging people sooner. It was easy for the HMOs to follow suit. Limiting procedures by requiring a pre-authorization became a standard procedure in the health insurance world.

Keep in mind, prior to the growth of HMOs, insurers just increased their rates when the costs increased and people seemed willing to pay. This was especially true because a fair degree of health insurance was paid for by employers. The government paid for Medicare, so why not? I used to say that in its early days, Medicare was a "pot of gold" that everyone just dug into to take out their share. That began to change in the 1980s and 1990s with the advent of DRGs and the growth of HMOs.

At Kaiser, it wasn't difficult for me to get involved with the hospital utilization management process. As a geriatrician, however, it wasn't about average length of stay numbers; it was about doing the right thing for each patient. We turned utilization management into discharge planning and called our daily hospital meetings care coordination rounds. We tried to make the process as interdisciplinary as possible. It was also my first foray into direct contact with other physicians regarding their approach to care. I often found myself asking them, on the fourth day of an admission, if they would hospitalize their patient if they had happened to see them in their office that day. The answer was invariably no. At the same time, I learned that we all develop habits and comfort zones and that changing those habits meant taking clinicians out of their comfort zone.

14.3 What About Geriatrics?

It's interesting that the field of geriatrics didn't take off in conjunction with this set of circumstances. We were in the right place, seemingly at the right time. I had joined Kaiser-Permanente. I had a few colleagues who had made similar moves. In the mid-1990s, several of us who were members of the American Geriatrics Society even started a managed care task force. What happened? Why didn't geriatrics take off? I believe that the reasons were complex. It certainly didn't help that there just weren't a lot of geriatricians around. In the early 1990s, a number of physicians grandfathered into their geriatric medicine board certification, but the number of physicians who had completed geriatric fellowships was quite small. Furthermore, most geriatricians lacked both training and experience in high level management, making it difficult for them to ascend the ranks. The few that did would ultimately run up against a traditional medical care culture that wasn't ready for the unique, and more holistic, approach that most geriatricians took. Finally, and for similar reasons, medical specialties, hospitals, and the pharmaceutical industry were absolutely not prepared for the high-touch, low-tech approach that I have spoken of in previous chapters. There simply did not appear to be a way to make a profit with the geriatric approach to care.

Despite all of this, we had developed an outpatient geriatric clinic at Kaiser. The first interesting phenomenon I noticed was that once our wait list was over 6 weeks, many of the patients that we had targeted would be admitted to the hospital prior to their first visit to us. We were definitely on to something! The adherence to our recommendations varied. In fact, while our clinic was inherently consultative in nature, some of the patients we saw ultimately just came to see us and we essentially took over their care.

14.4   Backlash Against HMOs

The other challenge in the 1990s in regard to managed care was the backlash against HMOs, made famous in the Jack Nicholson movie, "As Good as it Gets." Older adults were not signing up for HMOs in droves, which maintained the pressure for practices to survive in the fee-for-service model. I had moved to Denver in 1994 to join GeriMed of America, a geriatric medical management company that started out managing hospital-based senior health clinics. GeriMed's long-term strategy, however, was based on the core belief that managed care was the endgame. Ironically, we experienced the challenge of making this a reality when we tried to move all of our clinic patients from their fee-for-service-based Medicare insurance to a local HMO. Only about one fourth made the move, and we were ultimately forced to figure out how to survive in the fee-for-service world.

In 1989, MaxiCare, a large multistate HMO, declared bankruptcy. Its Medicare business was certainly a large part of their failure. In the mid-1990s, Oxford Health was the darling of Wall Street, promoting their innovative "disease management" programs, all of which seemed to save millions of dollars, while the company was losing millions. Chronically ill Medicare beneficiaries have multiple chronic diseases. A geriatric approach to their overall health would seem to make much more sense than multiple individual disease management programs. Or so it seemed to me at the time. With that said, there were attempts to bring geriatrics to the forefront of the managed care movement.

14.5   Exceptions to the Rule

There were exceptions to the lack of traction that geriatrics seemed to have in the 1990s. One of the first was On Lok, which was the first PACE (Program for All-inclusive Care of the Elderly) program in San Francisco. PACE is the program for patients who are eligible for admission to a nursing home, but are able to be maintained in a lower level of care. It combines the Medicare and Medicaid dollars that would normally be spent by the government for both medical care and housing. Another was Evercare, a United Healthcare product that brought geriatric nurse practitioners into the nursing homes. The Evercare program was even accompanied by some evidence-based research demonstrating its value.[1] The geriatric nurse practitioners were not hamstrung by productivity demands and were able to focus on the needs of the nursing home patients. I was also fortunate, in 1994, to join GeriMed of America. I have recounted our experience in the managed care realm in Florida in a previous chapter. Unfortunately, these programs were small exceptions to a very large rule. Geriatrics just did not take hold in the world of managed care in the 1990s.

It is worth noting that our experience at Senior Care of Colorado continued to be instructive between 2001 and 2010. While our practice operated on a fee-for-service model, half of our physicians were board certified and fellowship trained in geriatric medicine. Our nurse practitioners and physician assistants were trained in the geriatric approach to care. We ultimately participated in shared savings programs with our local Medicare HMO. Most importantly, having had access to the HMOs data, the fact that our providers were well educated in the geriatric approach clearly was conducive to a profitable business model. We had one of the lowest medical loss ratios in the community. Yet, we continued to be an exception to the rule.

14.6   Medicare Advantage

The Medicare Prescription Drug, Improvement, and Modernization Act of 2003 renamed Medicare HMOs as "Medicare Advantage" programs. Over the next 10 years, enrollment in these Medicare Advantage programs tripled to over 15 million enrollees. One of the problems with how the Medicare Advantage programs work is that historically high-cost geographic regions continue to provide far greater revenue to the insurance companies. It is not surprising that these areas tend to have higher penetration of Medicare Advantage programs. Rural areas, which historically have lower Medicare expenditures, provide lower payments to Medicare Advantage programs and ultimately tend to have fewer enrollees. With that said, the government has continued to try to encourage Medicare beneficiaries to join Medicare Advantage programs.

With the growth of Medicare Advantage programs has come attempts to make them more profitable. A lot of these efforts have focused on the "low hanging fruit," reducing hospital expenditures by shifting care and costs into skilled nursing facilities and home healthcare. Limitations on the choice of physicians have also accompanied this progression. The Centers for Medicare and Medicaid (CMS) have finally

---

[1] Kane RL et al. The effect of Evercare on hospital use. J Am Geriatr Soc. 2003 Oct; 51(10):1427–34.

tried to relate the quality of care to reimbursement, but the utility of existing quality measures as they relate to the care of older adults is still quite controversial.

As of late, we have also been seeing the consolidation of large insurers who provide Medicare Advantage programs. One has to wonder if this is a sign that the Medicare Advantage market feels that it has run out of ways to be profitable. Unfortunately, I believe this is because they have never been able to fully embrace many of the concepts that have been espoused in this book. If you are a geriatrician, and you know the way you practice, you have a full understanding of what I'm talking about. At the same time, you probably share my frustration regarding the willingness of the market to embrace the geriatric approach to care.

There are a few other beacons of light. Some of the insurers have begun to recognize the value of geriatricians and have been trying to incorporate them into their models. There are also pockets of practices that practice a geriatric approach that have been very successful working in partnership with a Medicare Advantage program. One of the greatest stumbling blocks to further growth in this area is the workforce. It is difficult to retrain practicing physicians in their approach to care. Finding and hiring the clinicians with the right skills has been a barrier for many of the successful practices that have worked in this space.

What does this all mean? Medicare HMOs have been pushed by the government for over 40 years. It seems that there are continued attempts to reinvent the managed Medicare wheel. Medicare HMOs, Medicare + Choice, and Medicare Advantage are all names for managed Medicare. We will discuss Accountable Care Organizations (ACOs) in a later chapter. One could argue that is not a very different model. Does repackaging mean that managed Medicare is dead? Or, does it mean that there will be continued attempts to find an acceptable Medicare Advantage model that works? Considering that I began my career with the belief that managed Medicare was the correct answer, I continue to hope for the latter.

14.7 Alternate Payment Models and the Future of Medicare Advantage

We will talk about alternate payment models in a later chapter, but the government is clearly attempting to reduce the Medicare program's reliance on fee-for-service reimbursement. This ultimately will further advance the development of Medicare Advantage and other managed care type programs such as ACOs.

Despite many studies to the contrary, everyone continues to push toward care coordination as the best model for approaching patients with multiple chronic diseases. The challenge has been in the integration of care coordination with the actual practice of medicine. This must be our future. Educating young physicians and reeducating the existing workforce to become competent in geriatric medical principles is ultimately the key to the success of Medicare Advantage programs.

Health systems that embrace the geriatric approach to care and an integrated care coordination model will be successful. Medical practices that do so have the potential to be successful as well. The challenge is finding a place where these entities can meet. As hospitals exist to provide acute care, the concept of empty beds, while logical, is foreign to those who own and operate hospitals. To the pharmaceutical industry, the concept of fewer medications is anathema to the bottom lines of the CEOs and shareholders. This is not an attack on the concept of profit motive and entrepreneurship in healthcare in general, but a recognition of the specific challenges in certain areas. The Affordable Care Act has attempted to address these issues, but in an albeit somewhat clumsy fashion.

There is a lot of discussion today about evidence-based medicine and value-based purchasing. What does that mean? To the frail older adult who is short of breath from congestive heart failure, and in pain from arthritis, this may not mean a longer lifespan. The field of palliative care has grown in leaps and bounds, but will soon hit the same brick walls that geriatrics has hit as it pushes on the profit margins of our traditional healthcare infrastructure. The growth of the alternative and complementary health industry should be a clear sign that the market place is struggling to deal with the traditional healthcare system. Still, for the individual, there will always be a place for western medicine.

Medicare Advantage still has an opportunity to be an avenue for the successful practice of geriatrics. Geriatricians must work to find common ground and to develop models of care that not only work for our patients but can fit hand in glove within a managed care approach. I believed that to be true nearly 30 years ago, and still believe it today. With that said, this is arguably the least optimistic chapter in this book. That is not meant to diminish our enthusiasm for the business of geriatrics, but to invigorate us to find ways of incorporating what we do best wherever the opportunity arises.

Business Planning for Geriatrics Success 15

If you're starting a practice or if you've been in practice awhile and need to go to a bank to borrow money, you're going to need to develop a business plan. When we decided to start Senior Care of Colorado in the winter of 2000, we actually had a very short timeframe in which to start our business. Since we were taking over a segment of an existing practice, there were some aspects that made this easier. On the other hand, the size of the practice presented immediate cash flow challenges. We needed to go to a bank and borrow money and obtain a line of credit. We needed a business plan. I didn't have any background in writing a business plan. I'd never taken a course in business.

15.1 Know How to Tell Your Story

What I did know was how to tell a story. I knew what we were trying to do. I also knew a lot about the market and the issues that we would be facing. Similarly, I'd been running a company and understood what a budget and balance sheet looked like. Now I just needed to translate what I knew to the written word. Following is the original business plan that we put together for Senior Care of Colorado in the winter of 2000. Not only is it still informative today, but can certainly be utilized as a platform for any geriatrics practice.

15.1.1 Senior Care of Colorado Business Plan: 2001

Senior Care of Colorado is a provider of services that focus on the medical care of older adults. Our core business is primary medical care for older adults in the outpatient, nursing home, hospital, and home settings. We also provide medical care for patients requiring skilled nursing care. We provide geriatric medical consultative services and specialize in evaluating and caring for older adults with memory impairment and dementia. Our physicians provide medical director services in

© Springer International Publishing Switzerland 2016
M. Wasserman, *The Business of Geriatrics*, DOI 10.1007/978-3-319-28546-7_15

nursing and assisted living facilities, as well as for hospice and home care agencies. Our physicians also act as expert witnesses in legal matters involving the care of older adults.

15.1.1.1 Mission

- To provide ready access to high-quality geriatric medical care in the community
- To offer expertise in the delivery of healthcare to older adults
- To provide a high level of customer service to our patients and clients
- To offer a work environment with the opportunity to achieve a high level of personal and professional satisfaction
- To educate the community on healthcare matters involving older adults

15.1.1.2 Business Model

Senior Care of Colorado is a professional corporation. Our bases of operations are two primary care physician office practices that focus on the care of older adults. One office is in Aurora, and the other office is in Downtown Denver. We presently provide medical care in over 20 nursing facilities in the Denver metropolitan area. Our physicians act as medical directors for several skilled nursing and assisted living facilities as well as some hospice agencies. Our physicians speak to professional groups and the community about geriatric medical care.

15.1.1.3 History/Background

The medical practices that are to be included in our business have been in existence in the Denver metropolitan area for several years. The offices in Aurora and Downtown were previously owned by Columbia/HCA and managed by GeriMed of America, Inc. In the spring of 1999, Rocky Mountain Geriatrics, PC (RMG), in conjunction with GeriMed, took over the office operations. Over the course of the following year, there was a determined effort to provide geriatric medical care in a global risk, managed care environment. This effort failed due to significant negative selection in an actuarially low number of patients. The partners in RMG have come to terms with GeriMed to fulfill whatever financial obligations resulted from this endeavor. Two of the RMG partners, Michael R. Wasserman, M.D., and Donald J. Murphy, M.D., decided to take over all existing operations and form a new corporation. All physicians in the present practice except for one have agreed to sign new contracts with Senior Care of Colorado. All existing staff has agreed to work for the new entity. Due to some changes in our focus, several employees have been laid off. We anticipate no further staffing changes at the present time.

Senior Care of Colorado will be utilizing GeriMed's electronic medical record (Care Management Software System™) that improves the quality of patient care and improves office efficiencies. We believe that this software also will help to maximize appropriate physician billing. The software program will be licensed from GeriMed for $1/year for the next 5 years. Our offices will function as beta sites for the further development of the software system.

15.1.1.4 Revenue
Our primary source of revenue is fee-for-service and capitated reimbursement for medical services. We have no existing contractual arrangements, nor do we plan to develop any, to take any financial risk for healthcare costs. Our secondary sources of revenue include payment for medical director and expert witness services. We also receive some revenue for speaking engagements and writing articles.

15.1.1.5 Expenses
The largest expense is for physician salaries. This typically accounts for 40–50 % of operating expenses. The next largest expense is for staff salaries. This typically accounts for 20–30 % of operating expenses. Remaining overhead expenses include office rent, equipment rental, office supplies, and utilities.

15.1.1.6 Staff
We will employ a total of nine physicians. The physicians will be paid based on a formula that provides them with a percentage of the actual revenue they are directly responsible for. This approach will minimize the greatest risk to a medical service business, that being decreased physician productivity. Any decrease in productivity and therefore revenue will result in a concomitant decrease in expenses. We will initially have 16 other employees. These include RNs, LPNs, medical assistants, and front office staff.

15.1.1.7 Benefits
We are presently awaiting a proposal. As the size of our company will allow us to use community ratings, we anticipate a decrease in the historical cost of health insurance for our employees. We do not plan on having a retirement plan in the year 2001.

15.1.1.8 Administrative Services
We are presently interviewing a couple of companies to provide accounting services. We will operate on a cash accounting methodology. We are also evaluating different payroll service companies to assist in the payroll function. We presently use an outside billing service to provide for the billing and collection for our medical services. They charge a fee of 8 % of collections. As primary care billing usually has a high volume of billing for relatively low amounts, bringing the billing function in house has significant risk with low potential yield. Nevertheless, we will continue to evaluate billing options.

15.1.1.9 Patient Base
Our Aurora office actively cares for over 2,200 Medicare beneficiaries. Our Downtown office actively cares for over 1,200 Medicare beneficiaries. Half of our outpatient population has Medicare plus a Medigap policy. The other half are members of the local HMO. We also care for over 1,000 patients in nursing homes and have a daily census of close to 50 patients at a skilled level of care in nursing facilities.

15.1.1.10 Revenue Projections

We have historical information on our existing practice. Due to the fact that the previous structure of the practices focused primarily on managed Medicare in a capitated environment, it is not accurate to utilize historical visit volumes. For example, under a capitated arrangement, many patient problems were addressed over the telephone and by ancillary staff. We have already begun to make a transition toward addressing patient problems with provider visits in the offices and the nursing facilities. We have also changed our visit times from 20 to 15 min per visit. This has been well received by our patients and has been achieved with no changes in staffing.

In Southeast Denver there is a paucity of physicians accepting patients with Medicare. A number of physicians have left the market and shut down their practices. As early as last week, another physician notified his patients that he was shutting his practice down. We anticipate continued high demand for the need for primary medical care services for older adults. Our focus and expertise has always led to a high degree of patient satisfaction.

15.1.1.11 Summary

Senior Care of Colorado is in the enviable position of having an existing patient base, offices, and full staffing. Our financial need focuses primarily on obtaining the necessary financial resources in order to cash flow the operation.

15.2 Be an Optimist

First of all, when you are preparing your business plan, you must be optimistic. As geriatricians, we tend to be realists and want to acknowledge the challenges as much as the potential successes. Banks want to know that you are aware of your challenges, but they also want to know the solutions that you are prepared to enact in order to be successful. Our meeting with the bank in December of 2000 had a positive outcome. We received a loan for $100,000 and took out a line of credit for $500,000. Having taken on an existing practice was helpful insofar as we were able to demonstrate a known revenue stream. Banks were also pretty favorable to loaning money to physicians at the time. Generally, so long as you can demonstrate that you understand both your revenue and expenses and that you expect to show a profit, banks will tend to respond positively to a physician practice.

At the end of the year, it is important to continue the narrative. It is a very valuable exercise and ultimately will prove important in regard to updating the business plan. Following is our end of year review from our first year of operations.

15.2.1 Senior Care of Colorado 2001 Highlights and Review

Our first year of operations proved both successful and exciting. From May through September, we averaged a net monthly profit of approximately $40,000. Consistent with that we were able to reduce our credit line from $415,000 to $273,000 during this time period. Reviewing our budget projections (calculated on an accrual basis) from 1 year ago, we had predicted revenues through September of $2,080,904 and expenses to be $1,963,249. Revenue, without including our expected A/R, was ahead of budget at $1,770,361. We have been very close to being on target with expenses of $1,937,025. Our collectable accounts receivable as of September 30 was $510,682, and as of October 31 was $620,098.

In September the opportunity to add an additional office, as well as a hospitalist function, presented itself. We agreed to integrate the practice of another physician at a third hospital. The long-term benefits far outweighed the short-term impact on cash flow. As we near year-end, the new office is almost fully integrated into our practice. Of note, our year to date expenses *include* some of the costs of absorbing the other doctors practice. The revenues *do not include* the addition of that practice and will add incremental revenue once our billing systems are fully in place by December of 2001.

Of note, Drs. Murphy and Wasserman, on advice from their accountants and attorneys, received an early dividend totaling $150,000 at the end of August. This was done to reflect their work efforts for the year prior to merging with the other doctors' practice. In order to do this, we needed to increase our credit line back to $423,000.

In November, the CEO of a Swedish hospital approached us about acquiring the assets of their busy senior clinic. While the hospital hasn't been successful (by their definition) in managing this practice, it has very similar characteristics to our Aurora office. Furthermore, there is a paucity of physicians accepting new Medicare patients in this part of town and a significant demographic need at the same time. We feel that this office can become a valuable part of our operation. We anticipate taking this practice on in either January or February of 2002. The fair market value of the assets of the practice should not exceed $75,000.

With our recent acquisitions, we have enhanced our position as the most substantial Medicare practice in Denver. Our expertise in geriatrics, including medical direction, has continued to garner us additional administrative work. We are presently in the early stages of developing a research arm, working with the pharmaceutical industry to perform clinical research. We believe that this can add further revenue to our bottom line. We also will be acting as expert speakers on a variety of geriatric topics, again bringing in additional revenue. Our role as expert witnesses in legal cases continues to grow.

In April we were fortunate to hire an outstanding practice manager, Ellen Springer-Jackson. Ellen brought considerable expertise in management and human resources. She has proven to be a stabilizing force in our practice as we have made numerous changes. In June we hired Shelly Thomas as both a site coordinator and billing/coding expert. Shelly has considerable experience in the area of billing and coding and will become our full-time billing manager and compliance officer when we bring billing in house early in 2002.

In September, realizing the extent of our growth and the increasing complexity of our operations, we engaged Steve Levey, of Gelfond, Hochstadt, Pangburn to assist us in improving our internal accounting functions. Mr. Levey also has extensive experience with other group practices here in Denver and has been very helpful in advising us on some of our recent business decisions.

We have seen very rapid growth this year and have no further expansion plans in the next 24 months. We plan to focus on systems and processes in order to further enhance our margin. One example of how we will continue to improve efficiencies this coming year is a plan to bring our billing process in house. This will improve customer satisfaction, patient residuals, and reduce cost. An expenditure of approximately $25,000 will be needed in order to capitalize the billing system. We anticipate annual savings of approximately $100,000.

There are three key elements responsible for our success. First, paying providers based on their production is a self-imposed insurance policy and has worked quite well. Only two providers have had trouble maintaining their salary level. Second, our electronic medical record, in addition to improving the quality of care we deliver, enhances our ability to code appropriately. Our average collection per office visit has proven to be substantially higher than first predicted, completely offsetting visit volume projections that were based on seeing more patients per hour than is reasonable in a geriatric practice. The final area has been office staffing, aided by the efficiencies of our computerized office systems.

The strength of our computer systems has led us to seriously consider linking all of our practices by way of a wide area network. This will require capital expenditures on the order of $50,000. We feel that the efficiencies gained will make up for the cost in fairly short order.

In order to complete our integration of the other doctor's practice, to capitalize the new practice at the Swedish hospital, and to enhance our computer systems, the three shareholders of Senior Care of Colorado, Drs. Wasserman, Murphy, and the third physician, would like to increase our existing personal loan of $100,000 to a loan of $300,000 at this time, payable over a 5-year period of time. We request that we maintain our line of credit at $500,000 at this time. Our early budget projections for 2002 suggest that we will continue to reduce our dependency on the line of credit as the year progresses.

15.3   Tying It Together

When looking back at our first year of operations, I would have to say that growing as fast as we did is not always advisable. However, opportunities arose and we chose to jump on them. While the bringing on of a third partner ultimately failed, the acquisition of a third clinic proved to be an important part of our future growth. I think that the important take-home point when it comes to business planning is that the story must make sense. It is critical that the bank see your business plan as both accurate and logical. It is actually okay to mention your challenges and problems, but should be able to explain how you successfully addressed dealing with them. With that history in mind, the business plan that we put together for the bank for 2002 follows. Take note that this plan drew significantly on the previous year's business plan but updated it where it was appropriate. It is always important for the story of the business to come across to the bank as continuous and seamless.

15.3.1 Senior Care of Colorado: 2002

Senior Care of Colorado is a provider of services that focus on the medical care of older adults. Our core business is primary medical care for older adults in the outpatient, nursing home, hospital, and home settings. We also provide medical care for patients requiring skilled nursing care. We provide geriatric medical consultative services and specialize in evaluating and caring for older adults with memory impairment and dementia. Our physicians provide medical director services in nursing and assisted living facilities, as well as for hospice and home care agencies. Our physicians also act as expert witnesses in legal matters involving the care of older adults.

15.3.1.1 Mission
- To provide ready access to high-quality geriatric medical care in the community
- To offer expertise in the delivery of healthcare to older adults
- To provide a high level of customer service to our patients and clients
- To offer a work environment with the opportunity to achieve a high level of personal and professional satisfaction
- To educate the community on healthcare matters involving older adults

15.3.1.2 Business Model
Senior Care of Colorado is a professional corporation. Our bases of operations are three primary care physician office practices that focus on the care of older adults. One office is in Aurora, another office is in Downtown Denver, and the third is at Rose Hospital. We provide medical care in over 30 nursing facilities in the Denver metropolitan area. Our physicians act as medical directors for numerous skilled nursing and assisted living facilities as well as some hospice agencies. Our physicians speak to professional groups and the community about geriatric medical care.

15.3.1.3 History/Background
Our medical office practices have been in existence in the Denver metropolitan area for several years. The offices in Aurora and Downtown were previously owned by Columbia/HCA and managed by GeriMed of America, Inc. In the spring of 1999, Rocky Mountain Geriatrics, PC (RMG), in conjunction with GeriMed, took over the office operations. Over the course of the following year, there was a determined effort to provide geriatric medical care in a global risk, managed care environment. This effort failed due to significant negative selection in an actuarially low number

of patients. Two of the RMG partners, Michael R. Wasserman, M.D., and Donald J. Murphy, M.D., decided to acquire the assets and form a new corporation as of January 1, 2001. In September we merged with a third doctor, who has an office and a very well respected hospitalist practice at another Hospital.

Senior Care of Colorado utilizes GeriMed's electronic medical record (Care Management Software System™) that improves the quality of patient care and office efficiencies. Our offices function as beta sites for the further development of the software system.

15.3.1.4 Revenue

Our primary source of revenue is fee-for-service reimbursement for medical services. We have no existing contractual arrangements, nor do we plan to develop any, to take any financial risk for healthcare costs. Our secondary sources of revenue include payment for medical director and expert witness services. We also receive some revenue for speaking engagements and writing articles.

15.3.1.5 Expenses

Provider salaries account for over 50 % of operating expenses. Staff salaries account for about 30 % of operating expenses. Remaining overhead expenses include office rent, equipment rental, office supplies, and utilities.

15.3.1.6 Staff

We employ a total of 11 physicians and 6 physician extenders. The physicians are paid based on a formula that provides them with a percentage of the actual revenue they are directly responsible for. This approach minimizes the greatest risk to a medical service business, that being decreased physician productivity. Any decrease in productivity and therefore revenue will result in a concomitant decrease in expenses. We have 30 other employees. These include administrators, RNs, LPNs, medical assistants, and front office staff.

15.3.1.7 Benefits

We offer competitive benefits through ADP TotalSource.

15.3.1.8 Patient Base

Our Aurora office actively cares for over 2,500 Medicare beneficiaries. Our Downtown office actively cares for over 1,200 Medicare beneficiaries. Our office at the other hospital cares for close to 1,000 patients. The patients do include some patients with commercial insurance. More than half of our outpatient senior population has Medicare plus a Medigap policy. The rest are members of Secure Horizons. We also care for over 1,300 patients in nursing homes and have a daily census of close to 50 patients at a skilled level of care in nursing facilities. Our hospitalist practice cares for an average daily census of 25 patients at the present time.

15.4 Using a Business Plan Template

It is notable how easy it is to use the basic template of one's business plan from year to year. It was not necessary to put in all of the details that had occurred so long as the ongoing business and budget made sense. Our next year was even more complex and ultimately required some good explanations. Our review of 2002 lays out what actually happened during the year. The act of writing an annual review is an excellent discipline to develop and will help you in planning for the upcoming year and beyond.

15.4.1 2002 Budget Review and Comments

Historically, Medicare office practices cannot support themselves due to high overhead and low revenue. As noted, a number of systems allow us to operate efficiently. We have continued to improve the effectiveness of our nursing home practice to include a nurse triage system that provides better care. It also helps to identify patients that need to be seen and providers who are available to see them in a timely fashion. The addition of a hospitalist function will further enhance revenues due to relatively low overhead. With Steve Levey's help, we anticipate improving our accounting systems to get a more accurate breakdown of our margins as they relate to the office, hospital, nursing home, home care, and administrative aspects of our practice.

The "Aurora and administrative" budget includes all corporate administrative overhead. We have a high level of confidence in our revenue and expense numbers based on last year's numbers. In addition, we will be actively educating patients and providers at all of our office on the use of our bone density machine, which Medicare covers in all older women every 2 years. The expected revenue for this is located under ancillary services. We have budgeted generously for outside accounting and legal services and hopefully will be able to reduce this number over the course of the year. Rent is increased for the extra administrative space we will be occupying. We also anticipate continuing to see 40–50 new patients, as we've been seeing monthly over the past year, and this will continue to allow our visit volume to increase.

We have adjusted our revenue per visit numbers to reflect actual experience and have chosen to be conservative with our figures. Historically, office revenue is between $92 and $96/visit and nursing home revenue is between $62 and $66/visit. Finally, we do expect an increase in revenue in speaking engagements, but have not included this in the budget.

We should see similar numbers at Swedish based on their historical experience. They already have a wait list for new patients and are located in an area of town with a paucity of doctors accepting new Medicare patients. We have not budgeted for an increase in patients or visit volume, which is conservative.

Our office at the other hospital has the fewest number of Medicare patients. Many of the hospital patients that we care for there do not have primary care physicians. We see this as an opportunity to increase our patient numbers. Furthermore, the other hospital is also limited in the number of primary care physicians accepting new Medicare patients.

Finally, we expect the Downtown office to show only a modest increase in patients and volume due to competition. The budget numbers are fairly easy to calculate based on previous experience at that location.

15.5   Fast Forward 6 Years

Six years later, our practice had continued to grow considerably. We had a few bumps on the road, some of which have been discussed in other chapters. I think that it is instructional that our business plan still followed the same format and continued to use much of the same language.

15.5.1 Senior Care of Colorado Business Plan (2008)

Senior Care of Colorado is a provider of services that focus on the medical care of older adults. Our core business is primary medical care for older adults in the outpatient, nursing home, assisted living, hospital, and home settings. We also provide medical care for patients requiring skilled nursing care. Some of our physicians provide medical director services for nursing homes and hospices. We provide geriatric medical consultative services and specialize in evaluating and caring for older adults with memory impairment and dementia. Physicians in our practice do a limited amount of speaking to other healthcare providers. Our physicians also act on occasion as expert witnesses in legal matters involving the care of older adults.

15.5.1.1 Mission
- To provide ready access to high-quality geriatric medical care in the community
- To offer expertise in the delivery of healthcare to older adults
- To provide a high level of customer service to our patients and clients
- To offer a work environment with the opportunity to achieve a high level of personal and professional satisfaction
- To educate the community on healthcare matters involving older adults

15.5.1.2 Business Model
Senior Care of Colorado is a professional corporation. Our bases of operations consist of three primary care physician office practices that focus on the care of older adults. One office is in Aurora, and the other two offices are in Englewood. We also have two satellite clinics in Westminister and Evergreen. We will be adding two more satellites this year, one in Centennial and the other in Louisville. We presently provide medical care in over 65 nursing facilities and more than 80 assisted living facilities. We care for patients as far south as Castle Rock, as far north as Greeley,

and as far west as Conifer. We also provide care to nursing facilities in Brighton, Fort Morgan, Brush, and Rifle. In addition, our providers perform visits in small group homes and in patient's homes. Our physicians also speak to professional groups and the community about geriatric medical care.

15.5.1.3 History/Background

The medical offices that are in our business have been in existence in the Denver metropolitan area for several years. The offices in Aurora and Englewood were previously owned by Columbia/HCA and managed by GeriMed of America, Inc. In the spring of 1999, Rocky Mountain Geriatrics, PC (RMG), in conjunction with GeriMed, took over the office operations. Over the course of the following year, there was a determined effort to provide geriatric medical care in a global risk, managed care environment. This effort failed due to significant negative selection in an actuarially low number of patients. The partners in RMG came to terms with GeriMed to fulfill whatever financial obligations resulted from this endeavor. Two of the RMG partners, Michael R. Wasserman, M.D., and Donald J. Murphy, M.D., decided to take over all existing operations and form a new corporation.

Senior Care of Colorado was formed in January of 2001. Initially, the office part of the practice consisted of the Aurora office and a Downtown office. In 2002 Senior Care of Colorado acquired the Englewood office from HealthONE while merging the primary care practice of Dr. Robert Leder. At the end of 2004, the Downtown office was closed and over 75 % of the patients being seen in that office were transferred to the other offices.

In 2006 we opened a satellite clinic on the campus of Covenant Village, a continuing care retirement community (CCRC) in Westminister. We also opened a satellite clinic in Evergreen, within a senior center run by Senior Resources, Inc, an organization that also provides for the transportation needs of the elderly in the community.

Senior Care of Colorado acquired the very highly respected nursing home practice of Dr. Robert McCartney in July of 2007. We also merged the primary care practice of Dr. David Palmquist on the Porter Hospital campus in December of 2007.

We have seen a fivefold growth in annual revenue since the inception of the company. We have doubled our number of providers in the past 2 years in preparation for handling what continues to be significant growth. Over the past 7 years, our practice has seen significant growth in terms of the number of nursing homes served. In the past 3 years, we have also seen a dramatic increase in the number of assisted living facilities where we deliver care. We have also seen an increase in our home visit program. In late 2006 we also began seeing our patients once or twice during their hospital stays. Our commitment to be with our patients "Every Step of the Way" has clearly spurred continued expansion and visit volume.

Senior Care of Colorado had previously used GeriMed's electronic medical record (Care Management Software System™) that improves the quality of patient care and improves office efficiencies. We have transitioned to software from SAGE, previously known as WebMD.

15.5.1.4 Revenue

Our primary source of revenue is fee-for-service reimbursement for medical services. We have fee-for-service contracts with EverCare, Secure Horizons, Rocky Mountain HMO, Humana, and Colorado Access. We have no existing contractual arrangements, nor do we plan to develop any, to take any financial risk for healthcare costs. We also receive some revenue for medical direction, speaking engagements, writing articles, and serving as expert witnesses.

15.5.1.5 Expenses

The largest expense is for provider salaries. This typically accounts for 50 % of operating expenses. The next largest expense is for staff salaries. This typically accounts for 25–30 % of operating expenses. Remaining overhead expenses include office rent, telephones, computer hardware and software, office supplies, and utilities.

15.5.1.6 Staff

We presently employ a total of 20 physicians and 28 physician extenders (physician assistants and nurse practitioners). We expect to add several more providers in 2008. They are all on salary and are eligible for bonuses based on productivity and other factors. We employ approximately 50 others. These include RNs, LPNs, medical assistants, billing clerks, and front office staff.

15.5.1.7 Patient Base

Our practice actively cares for over 11,000 Medicare beneficiaries. Sixty percent of our patient population has Medicare plus a Medigap policy. Ten percent have Medicare and Medicaid. Twenty-five percent are members of Secure Horizons, EverCare, Rocky Mountain HMO, or Colorado Access. We care for over 1,500 patients in over 65 nursing homes and have a daily census of over 300 patients at a skilled level of care in nursing facilities. Our practice averages 40–50 patients in inpatient settings across the Denver Metro area on any given day, making our group one of the largest inpatient admitters in the area.

15.6   Business Plans Tell a Story

This chapter is not only about how to write a business plan. *The story that is told is an experiential narrative that the reader may wish to read over a few times.* Some of the backstories have been shared in other chapters, but the flow of the development of our practice is informative in and of itself. Operating a geriatric practice is a dynamic and oft changing experience. There are many currents and eddies, and these must be navigated carefully. Mistakes will be made and, ultimately, it is not how many mistakes you've made, but how you react to them that matters the most.

They Don't Call It Risk for Nothing

16

Shared savings programs are one of the "alternative payment" methods that will purportedly revolutionize the Medicare program. When I hear and read this, I can't help but chuckle. In an earlier chapter, I shared a successful story about taking full risk with a Medicare population in Central Florida. There are certainly a number of successful examples of organizations and groups that have taken responsibility for the global Medicare dollars. I shared my experience with Kaiser Permanente, who clearly have demonstrated that taking risk on a large number of Medicare beneficiaries is possible, or not. Even Kaiser has had unsuccessful ventures into this arena. Similarly, at the same time that we entered into a full-risk relationship in Florida while I was at GeriMed of America, we contracted for a similar arrangement in Denver, Colorado. While we approached our patient population with the same model in Denver as we did in Florida, we were naive in regard to the demographics of our population. That naivete was deadly.

At the time that we entered into a full-risk Medicare contract in Denver, I was president and chief medical officer of GeriMed of America. I was also a member of Rocky Mountain Geriatrics (RMG), the physician group that GeriMed contracted with to provide care to the patients. For the prior few years, RMG had operated under a pure fee-for-service model within hospital-based senior clinics. However, when the hospitals had closed a number of these clinics, GeriMed proceeded to maintain a few of the clinics with the caveat that they would heavily market the patients to join the main Medicare HMO in the area. GeriMed negotiated a full-risk contract with the HMO. The members of RMG had agreed to share in the risk, and reward, with GeriMed. I was confident based on our experience in Florida as well as my belief in our model of care. Confidence is a double-edged sword when it comes to taking risk with a frail older adult population. If you are considering taking risk or entering into a shared savings program, read this chapter first!

117

© Springer International Publishing Switzerland 2016
M. Wasserman, *The Business of Geriatrics*, DOI 10.1007/978-3-319-28546-7_16

16.1 Actuaries Have Real Jobs

I never fully understood what actuaries did until I encountered the impact of not fully appreciating actuarial numbers. When we decided to sign a full-risk contract in Denver in the late 1990s, we didn't pay attention to the demographics of the patient base that we had been cultivating for many years. As our clinics had grown out of the hospital-based senior health clinic concept, we had drawn a population of patients who were in need of the services of geriatricians and a care coordination model. Our clinics had social workers who acted as care coordinators. Many of our physicians were board certified and fellowship trained in geriatric medicine. We didn't turn anyone down. No patient was too difficult, no family too demanding. It wasn't until 2000, when we put together an RFP for the Care Coordination Demonstration project, that it became obvious that close to 90 % of our patients fit the criteria for the project. While many practices complain that they have the sickest patients, we in fact did!

Most students of health policy today are aware that a fairly narrow band of the most frail Medicare beneficiaries are responsible for a large proportion of overall expenditures. Furthermore, actuaries will tell you that if you have fewer than 5,000 patients, the laws of chance put you in a very precarious position when it comes to actually impacting the overall cost of care. Both of these items were a double whammy to GeriMed and Rocky Mountain Geriatrics at the time that we entered into a full-risk contract with our local Medicare HMO. The results over the next year were instructive in many ways. The take-home lesson is that you should know as much as you can about the demographics of the population that you are about to go at full risk with. Actuaries are your best friend in this situation!

If you are entering a full-risk or shared savings model, it is critical that part of your due diligence is to fully evaluate the demographics of the population that you will be caring for. In today's healthcare world, there is plenty of data available to help one prepare for what they're getting into. The key term to be familiar with is the hierarchical condition category or HCC. This is how the government risk adjusts the payment allotted to Medicare Advantage programs. In preparing to care for a population, knowing the HCCs of that population will allow one to better judge their revenues. Similarly, knowing the types of chronic conditions that the patient population has will allow one to plan for the expected utilization of healthcare resources and services. Actuaries are our best friends under these circumstances.

16.2 They Don't Call It Risk for Nothing

When we took on the full-risk contract in Denver, there was no such thing as risk adjustment. We had a population of patients that were older and sicker than the average patient in the market. It should not be surprising that we got our butts kicked. We lost a ton of money (on paper) and had to go crawling back to the HMO in order to move forward with what ultimately became a pure fee-for-service practice. We had been so confident about our geriatric model and approach to care that we neglected the actuarial realities of the situation. One important lesson is that if you put all of your reimbursement at risk, you need to be prepared for the consequences. While shared savings models don't necessarily have the same downside risk as a full-risk arrangement, the potential impact on a practice that has a narrow margin can be just as devastating. I have to admit, we were not prepared and had to scramble quickly at the end to come up with a solution.

Not surprisingly, our greatest losses were in the realm of hospital expenditures. As I like to say, *numbers don't lie*. The Medicare program spends over 40 % of its annual dollars on hospital reimbursement. *If there's going to be a single facet of your program that loses the most money, look to your hospital utilization and costs first.* There is almost no reason not to look at hospital utilization first. There were some truly frightening aspects to our results. We had a couple of thousand of patients in the program and our portion of the losses was well into the six figure range. This was despite the fact that our hospital utilization was actually close to the community norm. However, we had self-selected the most frail members of our community. If a practice without care coordinators and geriatricians had taken risk on the same population, the losses for just a couple of thousand of patients would have easily been in the millions.

It was now clear that we could not sustain a full-risk approach to the patient population that we were serving. The losses sustained by GeriMed were manageable within the context of a larger corporate entity that could offset their losses in one market with profits from another market. From an actuarial context, this actually makes sense as well. Unfortunately, for RMG, as a small group of physicians, we were in a bind. None of the physicians involved had truly comprehended the impact of such losses. Something had to give. First of all, we had to come to grips with the fact that we could no longer take risk on our existing patient population. We also had to come up with a plan to move forward.

16.3 Negotiating to Survive

As president of GeriMed, and a member of Rocky Mountain Geriatrics, I was in a quandary. The other members of RMG had clearly had their fill of taking risk. As a company, it was clear to me GeriMed could no longer operate in the Denver market in the present situation. This was when Don Murphy made his fateful phone call to me that led to the formation of Senior Care of Colorado. We decided to make a go of a fee-for-service Medicare model, but first we had to get out from under the weight of the losses that we had incurred with our full-risk arrangement. Jim Riopelle, the CEO of GeriMed, brought us together for a meeting with the local Medicare HMO. They did not want to see our practice fold, as that would lead to the need to redistribute patients to other doctors in the market. They also understood that while we had lost money, we had lost far less than most community physicians would have lost under the circumstances. Ironically, we had actually saved the HMO a fair amount of money.

Negotiations are always an interesting experience. Even if you're in a weak position, you still have to look to your strengths. While our hospital expenditures had cost us money, we had actually profited when it came to our part B specialty costs. Geriatricians tended not to refer their patients out to specialists, and even with our high-risk population, we had held true to that. We explained to the HMO that we had done the best that we could have done under the circumstances. Unfortunately, our contract didn't give us the opportunity to obtain relief for doing our best. We had to live with the consequences of our full-risk contract. Still, we played the part of naive physicians, which in fact we had been, and suggested that unless the HMO provided some relief, we would be unable to continue the practice. As I had learned in Florida, HMOs were always sensitive to the issue of having adequate physician coverage for their patient population. If a practice folds completely, moving their patients, especially ones as complex and frail as ours, is not an easy task. Furthermore, mishandling that process can have costly consequences.

As president of GeriMed, I was in the awkward position of being on both sides of this equation. I also felt responsible for having gotten the physician group into the full-risk arrangement. Ultimately, we worked out an arrangement with GeriMed where the physician partners in RMG would take out a loan from GeriMed in order to pay their portion of the losses, and they would repay that loan over time. It was making the best of a difficult situation. We also negotiated a fee-for-service contract with the HMO so that we could continue to care for their patients in our remaining two clinics. RMG splintered further at the time and Senior Care of Colorado actually was born out of the ashes of our full-risk debacle. Life has an odd way of moving us forward. In fact, after this experience, only two of us felt comfortable taking the financial risk of starting a private geriatric practice.

16.4   Lessons Learned

It's very important when one takes risk to understand the population that you are caring for. Our failed experience occurred during a period of time prior to risk adjustment, which meant that our older and more frail population put us at a significantly higher actuarial risk of failure. Understanding actuarial risk is important, even if you are risk adjusted. The other aspect to this is to know the statistical risk of poor outcomes based on a relatively small sample size. Historically, it is common to take risk on Medicare populations of at least 5,000 people, although one can manage a smaller population if the risk adjustment dictates the possibility. However, one must recognize that a few outliers can skew your results. There are ways to protect oneself through stop-loss insurance and the like under these circumstances. Guessing is not the answer. Solid numbers are necessary in order to make rational decisions.

One of the other things that I learned is that it is important to understand your appetite for risk. It's also critical to know how your business partners feel. Physicians in general, and geriatricians in particular, are not risk takers. If one goes into a risk arrangement with partners who are risk adverse, poor decisions can ultimately be made in response to negative results. The other difficult factor is that as physicians, we have a responsibility, first and foremost, to the care of our patients. This responsibility cannot ethically be overtaken by business or financial needs. In the case of our situation, the partnership that RMG had with GeriMed allowed for some degree of a buffer. In the end, it was not enough. All of the physicians involved in this endeavor were certainly left with a negative feeling about the experience.

16.5   The Geriatric Approach Does Work

At the end of the day, despite the loss of money and the "failed" experience with a full-risk relationship, the data supported the geriatric approach and model of care. In fact, from the HMO's perspective, the model worked. At a time prior to risk adjustment, we had managed to significantly reduce utilization in a population that was presumably at the greatest risk. The problem for us was that the financial structure of the relationship was inadequate. With today's risk-adjusted approach, the exact same contract would have resulted in significant financial gain for all of those involved. Talk about being in the right place at the wrong time.

It is instructive, however, to review the results. First, the fact that specialty utilization and expenditures for such a frail, high-risk population was lower than expected speaks volumes about the model of care. In fact, despite our overall losses, we were actually profitable in this realm. Second, frail older adults will still end up with hospitalizations. Clearly, the importance of accounting for this with a risk adjusting methodology is necessary for a practice that is looking to put together a geriatric model. The other interesting lesson has to do with the fact that a geriatric practice will inevitably attract the more frail patients. This should not be surprising, and a risk-adjusted model can actually prove to be beneficial.

While it is instructive to recognize that the geriatric approach yields good results, it is also important to maintain some degree of caution when entering a risk relationship. A practice must understand its willingness to take risk, and it is very important to understand how the individual providers who are responsible for the care of the patients will react. There are a number of layers that need to be accounted for, but in particular, any individual that will be impacted by a negative outcome must be taken into account. The smaller the size of the patient population that risk is taken on, the greater the chance for an outcome that falls outside the law of averages. Taking risk is for real, and they truly don't call it risk for nothing.

ACOs: Days of Future Past

The Centers for Medicare & Medicaid Services (CMS) describes accountable care organizations (ACOs) as groups of doctors, hospitals, and other healthcare providers, who come together voluntarily to give coordinated high-quality care to their Medicare patients. ACOs have been a key element in the Affordable Care Act's approach in trying to reduce Medicare expenditures. On that level, they certainly deserve an entire chapter in this book. However, there is every reason for skepticism in relation to their efficacy in achieving such lofty goals. Recent results have already cast doubt on the ability of ACOs to truly be the future of Medicare. In fact, one has to question whether ACOs are truly a new idea or just another version of the HMOs of decades past.

The questionable value of ACOs doesn't preclude the significant opportunity that they bring to geriatricians and geriatric healthcare providers. For many of the same reasons that we discussed regarding how geriatric practices are tailor-made for a managed care setting, so too are they ideally aligned with ACOs. In fact, not only should geriatricians look for ways of working with ACOs, but the ACOs themselves should actively seek out geriatricians. Before we discuss this in further detail, it is worth looking at the types of ACOs that are out there.

17.1 ACO Models

Medicare offers a few different models for ACOs. The first is a Medicare shared savings program, where Medicare fee-for-service program providers have an opportunity to form an ACO. The second is an Advance Payment ACO model which is a supplementary incentive program for selected participants in the shared savings program. The third is the Pioneer ACO model, which was designed for early adopters of coordinated care.

CMS states that ACOs are not Medicare Advantage plans or HMOs. That is technically correct, but misleading from a practical perspective. Unfortunately, while ACOs have many of the same approaches and goals that managed care plans

© Springer International Publishing Switzerland 2016   123
M. Wasserman, *The Business of Geriatrics*, DOI 10.1007/978-3-319-28546-7_17

have historically had, they are without the means to operationally ensure that these approaches are routinely carried out. For example, the shared savings program has the following goals: better care for individuals, better health for populations, and lowering growth in expenditures. All of these are wonderful goals. How does a shared savings model help to bring these goals about? The apparent concept is that if incentives are aligned properly, then providers will do the right thing. HMOs and Medicare Advantage plans have a long history of offering similar shared savings models with their providers. Sometimes these are successful and sometimes they are not. Why are ACOs expected to have more success?

Into this chasm come opportunities for geriatricians to present themselves as solutions to the issues the ACOs will inevitably face. Since one of the challenges that ACOs have is the inability to require providers to practice in a way that meets the overall goals of the organization, utilizing geriatricians and geriatric practices at key points along the continuum actually presents a firewall of sorts in regard to some of the issues that have historically plagued managed care companies. One of the first points of contact that has the greatest impact on Medicare expenditures is the acute care hospital.

17.2 Hospitals Are Incentivized to Admit

One of the major challenges that ACOs face stems from the fact that they are often led by hospitals or hospital-laden health systems. Historically, hospitals earn a living by filling their beds. While the concept of making money by reducing hospitalizations may theoretically sound good even to a hospital, on a practical level it is very difficult to achieve. There are multiple reasons for this, the least of which is that the hospital will continue to fill its beds with non-ACO patients as well, setting up the potential dichotomy of treating two patients with the same condition in a different manner. There is also the issue of inertia. It is hard to change the practice pattern of clinicians, especially if the incentives are not entirely clear, which in the frail elderly is likely to be the case.

The results from the first 2 years of the Pioneer ACO experience demonstrated some net savings, but many of the programs were unsuccessful. This begs the question regarding implementing a program that is not routinely successful. We cannot afford to institute methods that only work half the time and with half the providers. Digging deeper into the cost savings, one typically finds savings primarily in the hospital realm. This is not surprising in terms of the "low-hanging fruit" that is clearly available when it comes to the historical approach to caring for older adults which brings us back to the question of how to deal with the acute hospital in the setting of an ACO.

What tends to stand out among the ACO experiment is that yet again there has been little focus on the geriatric approach to care. Combined with the paucity of geriatricians and providers who are competent in geriatric medicine, it is not surprising that the national results have been mixed. For this reason, ACOs should be aggressively looking at how to bring the geriatric approach to care into the acute hospital setting. One of the simplest ways is with an Acute Care of the Elderly (ACE) unit. ACE units have the effect of "geriatricizing" the acute hospital setting. Not only have such units been shown to reduce hospital length of stay but they have also been shown to reduce readmissions.

17.3   The ACE Opportunity

The inertia of the acute care hospital runs counter to the geriatric approach to care. High touch and low tech are not typical bywords of acute care. Sometimes, aggressive and high-tech care are necessary in the treatment of frail older adults. But oftentimes, less is more. Furthermore, once a frail older patient has turned the corner, there often needs to be an aggressive switch to a more traditional geriatric model of care. This type of approach is clearly in the wheelhouse of an ACE unit.

Politically, building an ACE unit within a hospital means going up against the established approach to care of the other medical and surgical specialties. Since most hospitals continue to provide care to fee-for-service patients, they are in a quandary. Do they ruffle the feathers of the interventionists? Do they shy away from the higher revenue, procedure-laden approach? Ironically, one of the differences that ACOs have from more traditional managed care structures is that it is the fee-for-service patients themselves who will ultimately impact the ACO's bottom line.

At the very least, an ACO should look for a geriatrician to provide leadership in their organization. Out in the marketplace, a geriatric practice should aggressively seek out their local ACO. They can provide solutions to issues that the ACO may not often fully appreciate. Helping to build and staff an ACE unit provides a win-win situation for a geriatric practice. From a very practical perspective, it provides work for the practice. Additionally, it provides a direct connection to patients who will require skilled nursing care after discharge. Since SNF care should be an integral part of a geriatric practice, this becomes an important strategic opportunity.

17.4   The "Black Hole" of SNFs

Hospitals generally don't have a clue when it comes to dealing with skilled nursing facilities. Emergency room physicians often see nursing homes as places where older patients are neglected. Hospitals haven't moved very far past this level of understanding. While they recognize the need for nursing facilities when it comes to discharging patients, they don't necessarily appreciate the care that can be provided along the long-term care continuum.

Ironically, the skilled nursing homes see the hospitals as necessary evils in their own survival. They depend upon the hospital for admissions, but they complain and struggle with patients being sent to them with inadequate information and expensive (and often unnecessary) medications. They are also quite aware of how the emergency room and hospital view them, which creates an environment of mistrust and disrespect. This quagmire creates another opportunity for geriatricians, who are generally experienced and well trained in the culture and workflow of skilled nursing facilities.

There is a huge differential in the expenditures an ACO has between hospitals and skilled nursing facilities. Most approaches that aim to reduce hospital costs will inevitably result in shifting care into nursing facilities. Similarly, there are already ongoing efforts in the fee-for-service arena to reduce readmissions from skilled nursing facilities back to the acute hospital. The black hole that is the skilled nursing facility can quickly become the focal point for reducing costs.

17.5 Direct SNF Admissions

Everyone involved in caring for Medicare patients knows about the "two midnight" rule. A Medicare patient must be in the acute hospital for three days in order to qualify for a skilled nursing facility stay that is covered by Medicare. This rule was put into place to avoid the presumed abuse of skilled nursing, which is somewhat ironic when one compares the cost of a skilled nursing day to an acute hospital day. Furthermore, it is unlikely that patients and families would willingly abuse this opportunity as well. In fact, at the end of the day, this rule may have inadvertently encouraged acute hospital stays in order to get patients into a skilled nursing opportunity. While CMS has not changed this rule, managed care companies have long had the ability to ignore it. Back in the late 1990s, GeriMed of America took advantage of this opportunity in both the Denver and Florida markets. We developed relationships with skilled nursing facilities where it was possible to admit a Medicare Advantage patient directly to the skilled nursing facility and bypass the hospital. EverCare similarly had a reimbursement methodology that allowed for higher acuity services for residents of long-term care facilities in lieu of the need for an acute hospital admission.

For many frail older adults, a direct admission to a skilled nursing facility can actually be the most appropriate care approach. First of all, skilled nursing facilities often have staffs that are more attuned to the needs of the frail older adult. Second, there is often an immediate focus on rehabilitation that often doesn't exist in the acute hospital setting. Third, it is clearly the least expensive level of care. A direct admission would not be appropriate for a patient who requires an intensive care unit level of care, but many frail older adults don't need that level of care and often don't want that level of care. Pioneer ACOs have actually had the opportunity to apply for a waiver from the 3-day stay rule. In order to have a waiver granted, it is necessary to demonstrate the type of a systematic approach to such patients that a geriatric practice is most suited to provide.

17.6 An Opportunity to Build the SNF Relationship

One of the major things that a direct SNF admission program offers is an opportunity to further develop the relationship with the skilled nursing facilities themselves. The geriatrician and the geriatric practice are actually well positioned to facilitate this relationship. Furthermore, if there is a medical director relationship involved, there is a further opportunity to improve the educational focus of the facility in order to enhance the type of care necessary for such programs to work.

If there is an ACO in the area, it behooves a geriatric practice to become involved. Not only are they positioned to provide a bridge to the skilled nursing facilities but clearly have an opportunity to both improve care, while providing what tends to be a more cost-effective approach. The geriatric practice will also be seen as bringing value to the skilled nursing facilities at the same time. It is always good to look for win-win opportunities in the marketplace! Skilled nursing homes are all about relationship building, and they are certainly living in the eye of the ACO "storm."

17.7   Delivering Consistent Care

It should not be surprising that it is possible for two patients with the same clinical conditions might receive varying degrees of care despite sharing a room in a skilled nursing facility. This has long been an issue in regard to different payment sources. For example, a resident who has fee-for-service Medicare with a Medigap plan will typically receive more skilled nursing days than a similar patient who is part of a Medicare Advantage program. The number one difference has to do with how the care of the individual is coordinated and who holds the purse strings.

A geriatric practice has as its fundamental principle the goal to provide quality care to its patients. Clinical decisions should be based on what's best for the patient. In the acute hospital setting, this often means discharging the patient as soon as is humanly possible. Hospitals have plenty of potential iatrogenic complications to make prolonged stays undesirable. Similarly, patients who are receiving skilled nursing care in a SNF should aspire to be discharged home as quickly as possible. At the present time, however, many skilled nursing facilities benefit from a longer stay, as this keeps higher revenue beds filled.

ACOs will have to grapple with the overall cost of care that their patients receive and once again their ability to control SNF length of stay will be recognized as an important approach to reducing overall costs. How will they accomplish this? They may try various means to accomplishing this end, but are best suited to engaging facilities through providers who can deliver a geriatric approach to care. Hence, geriatricians and geriatric practices find themselves at the heart of this relationship.

It is critical that the geriatric practice has a singular approach to care in the nursing facilities they attend. The first and foremost reason has to do with the concept of quality and consistency. From a clinician's perspective, being asked to take different approaches to similar patients is not a healthy environment to practice in. The ethical ramifications are questionable as well. Similarly, as we have discussed many times in the pages of this book, the geriatric approach to care tends to be cost-effective. This aligns the clinician well with the ACO while at the same time delivering care that patients and families will ultimately appreciate.

17.8   Seize the Day!

While accountable care organizations have a multitude of challenges ahead of them, it appears that CMS is fixated on utilizing them as a means toward overall reduction in Medicare expenditures. Quality measures, however tenuous in the frail elderly population, will also be an important aspect of ACOs. Into this vortex comes an opportunity for geriatricians and geriatric practices alike. We can sit around the doctor's lounge and whine about how the government is ruining healthcare by intruding on our livelihoods, or we can seize the day and offer our expertise and services. This is clearly an area that those with a knowledge of geriatrics and the continuum of care can shine. For all of the challenges that ACOs may encounter in affecting the care of older adults, we may be the ultimate solution!

Bundling and Alternate Payment Models 18

The future of Medicare is sprinkled with the promise of Alternative Payment Models (APMs). The general idea is that the traditional fee-for-service reimbursement model isn't working. Although they are interesting, the reason for this isn't the focus of this book or this chapter. The general idea of APMs is that they fulfill a couple of key functions. As Medicare struggled to impact the ongoing growth of its expenditures, one of the approaches is to find ways to put a cap on physician spending. The previous attempt at doing so, which was related to the SGR, led to annual battles between physicians and congress. That has been "fixed," and in its place are alternatives that we will discuss shortly. Alternative payment approaches have also been linked to the concept of value and improving quality.

One of the latest approaches in this attempt to rein in Medicare expenditures is the concept of "bundled payments." The idea is that a set payment for an episode of care will incentivize healthcare providers to be conscientious about the cost of the care that they provide. While we could spend this entire chapter discussing what is potentially wrong with this approach, it is once again important to view the incredible opportunity that exists for geriatric healthcare providers.

18.1 Right Place at the Right Time

When it comes down to it, many of the bundled payment programs attempt to achieve their success primarily by reducing hospital admissions or readmissions. This should sound familiar by now, as should our response to this approach. The geriatric approach to care within a geriatric model of care will win the day most every time! Geriatric practices are poised to help assure the success of bundled payment models. The first step along the way is our relationship with and skills within the long-term care continuum. Using skilled nursing, assisted living, and home visits as tools to avoid hospitalization in the setting of certain chronic diseases is definitely in the wheelhouse of geriatric healthcare

© Springer International Publishing Switzerland 2016
M. Wasserman, *The Business of Geriatrics*, DOI 10.1007/978-3-319-28546-7_18

providers. We discussed many of these principles in the chapter on accountable care organizations.

Similarly, bundled payment programs for procedures that occur in the hospital setting, such as total hip and knee replacements, are a natural setup for a geriatric practice to reduce readmissions. While it might seem to outside observers that the place for the geriatrician is just in the skilled nursing facility, the opportunity is across the entire continuum. This concept needs to be sold to whomever is responsible for the bundled payment.

18.2   Outpatient Geriatric Consultation: Preparation!

Waiting until the procedure is performed without preparing beforehand misses the opportunity to reduce the risk of complications from whatever procedure is to be performed. Outpatient geriatric consultation provides ample opportunity to evaluate and prepare the patient for what is to come. *A full evaluation of the patient's medications by a geriatrician will allow for the reduction or discontinuation of unnecessary or potentially harmful medications.* There might also be the opportunity to suggest physical or occupational therapy prior to the procedure itself. Finally, a full evaluation of the patient's social circumstances, integrated into the medical evaluation, will identify potential pitfalls that are often missed by the traditional approach to care.

A geriatric practice will need to navigate the politics of providing geriatric consultation in the community. If the practice also delivers primary care services, this will be a very important issue to address. Other primary care physicians in the community might feel threatened by the fact that their patient is being seen by another primary care physician. This can usually be dealt with strategically. First, the more complex the patient, the less likely it will be that their primary care physician will be threatened by a geriatrician's evaluation of their patient. Oftentimes, these patients are time consuming to the primary care physician, who may actually see such a patient as a drain on their practice's resources. Furthermore, if the primary care physician ultimately gains some financial benefit from the success of the bundled payment model, then having their patient seen by a geriatrician might be acceptable. There are clearly a lot of moving parts in such a scenario, which means that it is also just as likely that whomever is responsible for the bundled payment might not be paying attention to all of the political intrigue that might develop in the physician community.

If you have an outpatient practice in a community that is involved in a bundled payment program, it behooves you to identify your practice to those who hold the purse strings for the program. Making a business case for why an outpatient geriatric consultation will ultimately save money is an opportunity that must be taken. At the same time, the community dynamics and politics will often require co-opting the leadership of the bundled payment program. It is important that they be on your side when selling your involvement in the program to the rest of the medical community.

18.3 Promoting Our Experience

Many geriatricians have spent their careers hearing other clinicians question our approach to care. They often will point out that we don't have "data" or evidence to support many of the approaches that we take. Whether it's outpatient geriatric consultation or reducing medications, we will often be placed on the defensive by specialists who insist that their methods are better than ours. This is an area where we must not be shy! Those of us who have practiced geriatrics for many years have a collective experience with a significant "n" attached to it. While there may not be specific data to the precise issue that we are engaged in at a given moment, there is definitely a growing body of data on the value of the geriatric approach to care. Furthermore, it is also okay to respond to such critiques by pointing out that the "acceptable" approach is also lacking in data and evidence. Combining this with specific experiential examples, as well as comparisons such as those noted in our chapter on geriatric medicine, is the ammunition that geriatricians have in order to defend themselves from such attacks.

It's also important to remember the importance of the patients and their families when suggesting what might seem to be a less "conventional" approach to care. One of the great things about the geriatric approach is that it has a lot of common sense attached to it, which makes it very amenable to explaining to non-clinicians. The average person tends to understand that hospitals are dangerous places (even hospital administrators!). No one really wants to take lots of medications, and everyone has an experience with an older loved one when it comes to an adverse reaction to a medication. These experiences can be used to our advantage when promoting our approach to care. Similarly, anecdotes can have meaning when they make sense and they can be supported with years of experience. Finally, and this suggestion is worth repeating, *when others ask us for data on the value of our approach to care, it is entirely reasonable to request similar data on their approach.* There will often be none!

18.4 Inpatient Geriatrics: Clinical Management

In the previous chapter, we discussed the value of an Acute Care of the Elderly (ACE) unit in the setting of an ACO. Such a unit would also be useful in a bundled payment model. With that said, there are not a lot of ACE units at this time, and as we discussed, there is a fair amount of political maneuvering that is required to put one in place. An inpatient geriatric consultation program might have to suffice as the best means of injecting the geriatric approach to care into the bundled payment care process. Again, while this might prove to be a singular opportunity for a geriatrician or geriatric practice, it also could be an excellent chance for a geriatric practice to insert itself into the entire process. As noted in the last chapter, the geriatric practice can also leverage its knowledge of and relationship with skilled nursing facilities to improve care outcomes after discharge.

An inpatient geriatric consultation service should not function with a geriatrician alone. Geriatrics being an interdisciplinary process requires other team members in order to achieve the most effective results. At a bare minimum, a geriatric nurse specialist should be involved in the team. Ideally, a social worker should also be a team member, but if resources are short, the nurse specialist can usually provide an adequate skill set in regard to care coordination. If possible, a geriatric pharmacist can provide a significant added resource and extend the reach of the geriatrician.

Determining how the practice will be reimbursed will ultimately decide who employs the rest of the team. In an ideal situation, the practice will have negotiated a set fee for the entire team's services, or a piece of the shared savings in the bundled payment model. Some of this will depend on the level of risk aversion that the practice has. *It is always ideal for all of the team to be employed by the practice.* Having team members who are employed by the hospital sets up potentially challenging management dynamics.

With that said, if employing the nurse specialist or social worker is not possible, then the practice should require that the hospital provides the staff. Operationally, this will create new problems, but without the other team members, the effectiveness of the geriatrician will be limited. Nevertheless, both patients and other clinicians involved in the care of the patient should find the inpatient geriatric team to be a useful adjunct.

18.5 Geriatrics Along the Continuum of Care

Potentially, the most important realm in the mission to reduce the risk of a hospital readmission is along the continuum of care. As discussed in other chapters, the nursing home setting provides the most obvious example, but assisted living facilities should not be ignored. Finally, a robust home visit program can be very useful regardless of whether the patient enters a skilled nursing facility. The geriatrician clearly lives and works in this realm, making this a substantial opportunity for a geriatric practice.

There are a myriad of opportunities available for geriatricians in relation to caring for the patients in skilled nursing facilities. A robust SNF program allows for daily follow-up of patients and will reduce anxiety in relation to an early discharge from the acute hospital. There is no question that daily follow-up and the ability to address acute problems in the SNF 24 h a day, seven days a week is paramount to preventing readmissions to the hospital. Furthermore, the geriatrician also provides a necessary bridge for effective clinical communications with the SNF.

Another opportunity in regard to impacting the care along the continuum is for the geriatrician to engage in their role as a nursing facility medical director. This position allows the geriatric practice to lead the approach to care from within the care continuum. Communications between the hospital and skilled nursing facility are critical and require facilitation with which the medical director can be instrumental. There is a fair amount of distrust that presently exists between acute hospitals and skilled nursing facilities. If this is not dealt with effectively, the long-term success of a bundled payment program could easily be in jeopardy.

18.6   The Pay's the Thing

All of the aforementioned thoughts are useful, but from a practical perspective, how the geriatric practice fits into the payment scheme is of high importance. In many of the bundled payment model programs, providers are paid their typical fee-for-service reimbursement. After the episode of care is complete, there is a reconciliation of all of the Medicare expenditures, and there is either net savings or loss. If there is savings, the party responsible for the bundled payment program will receive a bonus; if there is a loss, the amount will be recouped from future reimbursements. There is also a bundled payment model where a prospective payment is made to the hospital, and they are responsible for paying the providers.

Understanding the payment methodology is important for many reasons. First and foremost, if the practice is providing services, it is critical that the practice's reimbursement adequately covers the cost of those services. If there are to be bonuses, a system for aligning incentives needs to be developed in advance, and it must make practical sense. If the hospital receives a prospective payment, then there needs to be a contractual arrangement between the geriatric practice and the hospital that delineates the services that will be provided and how they will be paid for. This is a unique opportunity to build a team-based approach and have it paid for. What the practice must be cautious of is not to provide services that are labor intensive that do not come with adequate reimbursement. There may also be an opportunity to take risk and share in the savings with the hospital. Understanding the formulas and calculations for such a program are very important.

Physicians are not typically trained in developing financial modeling, nor in the art and science of negotiating. There are a lot of moving parts in bundled payment programs, and therefore a lot of opportunities for both revenues and expenses. A geriatric practice must put all of the work that will be performed on the table. This may include everything from outpatient and inpatient consultation to an SNF and home visit program. It is important to literally put together a business plan for such a program and to critically review every aspect.

Bundled payment plans provide an incredible opportunity for geriatricians and geriatric practices, but are also filled with land mines that can lead to financial losses if the practice is not careful. There is a fair amount of money out there, but it can get chewed up quickly along the continuum. Clearly, the hospital is the most likely place for the money to be spent, and the overhead inherent in hospitals can add up quickly. Taking as much of the bundled payment process out of the hospital is the quickest way to reduce overall expenditures, but will be a challenging task as historically this is where most of the money goes. While this is a consistent theme, yet again it must be looked at as an opportunity rather than an impediment.

18.7   Other Alternative Payment Models

There are presently other alternative payment models that are planned for physicians to be able to work with, and there will certainly be additional models that come forth. Many of these models are variations on similar themes that we have and will address in this book. They include the shared savings model and accountable care organizations. There are also primary care and medical home-related models. All of these models have a commonality when it comes to the need to provide efficient, high-quality, and cost-effective care to frail older adults. They are all opportunities for geriatricians and a geriatric practice!

MIPS and Geriatrics

<big>**19**</big>

Incentivizing physicians to deliver quality care has become the Holy Grail of healthcare. To be completely fair, the driving force in the development of quality measure and performance improvement has been the desire to lower Medicare expenditures. Thus, there will generally be a direct relationship between the program and reimbursement. In a fee-for-service environment, this occurs at the point of physician reimbursement. In an alternative payment model, it may ultimately be reflected by a shared savings model.

The Centers for Medicare & Medicaid (CMS) have a recent history of trying to develop performance improvement incentives for physicians. The Physician Quality Reporting System (PQRS) program was their first major attempt to encourage improved quality of care through both incentives and penalties. This program is now going to be absorbed by something called the Merit-Based Incentive Payment System (MIPS). It is not our intent to go into specific detail on a program that will not be rolled out for a couple of years, but rather to describe the basic principles necessary for a geriatric practice to engage and address such programs.

Our experience with incentive-based programs has been fairly robust, from an internal perspective both dealing with individual clinicians and dealing with incentive programs brought forth by both managed care entities and CMS. In the spirit of learning from our experience, let's start by looking at how our practice at Senior Care of Colorado approached the PQRS issue when it first arose.

19.1 Time Is Money

The first thing one has to do when posed with a new pay for performance methodology is to analyze its impact on your practice. The simplest example is that if the systems that need to be put in place increase practice expenses or reduce the practice's revenues by 10 %, then a five percent incentive does not work! Many practices have learned this the hard way, wondering why they are losing money despite getting "bonus" payments. The reality is that "time is money." At the end of the day,

© Springer International Publishing Switzerland 2016
M. Wasserman, *The Business of Geriatrics*, DOI 10.1007/978-3-319-28546-7_19

whether one is in a fee-for-service environment or not, practice revenue and expenses are definitely impacted by how many patients can be seen in a day.

The productivity aspect of revenue is pretty obvious. Oftentimes, the more patients seen in a day, the greater the revenue. Other things being equal, such as the billing codes remaining the same, a decrease in the number of patients will result in less revenue. The expense side is less obvious. In a capitated environment, where it might not seem to matter how many patients an individual provider needs to see in a day, the ability of the practice as a whole to care for all of the patients is paramount. Productivity does matter in this environment, because a reduction in a provider's efficiency will result in the practice needing to hire more providers to manage the clinical demand. This results in an increased expense to the bottom line. On the other hand, in a shared savings environment, the extra time spent by a clinician could ultimately lead to bonuses that pay for that additional time. The ultimate answer will become obvious in the profit and loss statement of the practice!

A red flag should come up when the mechanics of documenting for pay for performance measures takes valuable direct patient care time away from a clinician. The PQRS system has had this impact on practices by distracting clinicians from their usual documentation patterns. This is a challenge that should never be discounted. In fact, recognizing the challenges is the first step in embracing pay for performance opportunities.

19.2   Incorporating Pay for Performance into Workflow

Regardless of the criteria being accounted for in a pay for performance model, the ability to track the data defines ones' chance of being rewarded for a particular result or behavior. In the age of electronic health records, most of this information will be available electronically. As a wise computer programmer once told me, "computers are dumb as posts." The validity of the data is only as good as the human beings who input that data. The PQRS program required various processes and outcomes on the part of a medical practice. Was a patient given tobacco cessation information? Was their Hemoglobin A1C below a certain level? Were patients offered, and did they receive their influenza vaccine?

Theoretically, some of the data can be collected through actual claims, which at the very least requires appropriate coding and billing by the clinician or the practice. In fact, historically, there have been codes corresponding to the specific PQRS items that need to have been documented in the medical record. With the advent of more sophisticated electronic health records, it has been possible for a clinician to check off a box in their progress note that directly links to the corresponding billing code. This highlights the importance of looking at workflow dynamics in relation to pay for performance incentives.

One of the less understood aspects of requiring specific elements of data entry is the impact that documenting those elements has on the clinicians train of thought and documentation patterns. To a computer programmer, this may not seem to matter, but anything that interrupts the clinician's flow of thinking has the potential of prolonging the time of the visit. One to two minutes per patient over the course of a day can equal the time it takes to see one to two more patients. This has the potential of reducing productivity by five to ten percent. If the penalty for not complying is less than five percent, we have a conundrum. We should also not discount the potential impact on quality of care that distractions from a clinician's normal way of thinking might pose. When dealing with the frail elderly, the impact of each instance could have a geometric effect on decision-making!

The ideal situation for tracking the necessary data elements is to incorporate the information necessary for compliance with incentive programs into the natural flow of a patient visit. For example, when documenting a patient's smoking history, the opportunity to capture whether advice regarding smoking cessation was given should be readily available. In an ideal future world of electronic health records, the discussion that the physician has with the patient regarding their smoking habits and recommendations to stop smoking will be captured by voice recognition software and automatically fed into whatever tracking mechanism exists in the program. Similarly, when discussing health prevention, assuring that a patient has received or been offered their influenza vaccine fits neatly into a routine visit while capturing a key data element for compliance with a pay for performance program.

19.3   Choosing the Appropriate Measures

As the above examples suggest, it makes sense for the practice to monitor and report on measures that fit best into the flow of a clinician's visit. They should also have the most pertinence for the population that the practice cares for. The example of monitoring influenza vaccination status certainly makes a lot of sense in the frail elderly. On the other hand, very few 95-year-olds are still smoking, so that metric may be of much less value and importance.

It is often a good idea for the practice to put a focus group of clinicians together to discuss the best measures to focus on. Such discussions should include getting input from the clinicians in regard to how they will fit the pertinent questions into their exam. If the practice has particular templates, this would be a great time to look at how those templates might be adjusted to allow for the collection of the necessary data elements that will correspond to the identified quality measures.

With this in mind, PQRS has been the focus of most practices in recent years. This focus is about to change, although the specifics will undoubtedly change in the coming years. With change ahead, we need to pose the question of what we have to look forward to with the MIPS program as it has been proposed.

19.4   What's Ahead?

The Merit-Based Incentive Payment System (MIPS) is scheduled for roll out in 2019. It is never too early to start preparing for programs such as this. In fact, with penalties beginning in 2019, it is quite likely that performance from 2017 will be evaluated. Thus, practices should start working now on developing systems that fit into their workflow. Existing penalties in the PQRS program will actually sunset at the end of 2018. However, PQRS will not completely go away. The new MIPS program will actually combine the existing PQRS program with meaningful use (MU) and a value-based payment modifier (VBPM) into a single program. The program is based on performance in four categories: quality, resource use, clinical practice improvement activities, and meaningful use of an electronic health record system. Beginning in 2019, physicians will be eligible for both positive and negative Medicare payment adjustments that start at 4 % and increase to 9 % by 2022.

There will be an interesting alternative to the MIPS program. Practices will have the opportunity to be part of an alternative payment model (APM). Initially, there will be three pathways for a practice to take: Accountable Care Organizations (ACOs), which include the Pioneer ACO program and the Medicare Shared Savings Program; Bundled Payment Programs; and payment models tied to patient-centered medical homes. The future will certainly bring additional alternative payment models, but the concepts should remain the same. There will also be a timeline by which the practice receives an increasing proportion of its revenue through such alternative models.

19.5   Clinical Practice Improvement Activities

The MIPS program will focus on a set of clinical practice improvement activities.

While these are yet to be fully defined and will be developed by CMS's usual approach of sharing with the public and asking for comments, there are some examples that have already been shared. These include the following[1]:

1. Expanded practice access, such as same day appointments for urgent needs and after hours access to clinician advice
2. Population management, such as monitoring health conditions of individuals to provide timely healthcare interventions or participation in a qualified clinical data registry
3. Care coordination, such as timely communication of test results, timely exchange of clinical information to patients and other providers, and use of remote monitoring or telehealth
4. Beneficiary engagement, such as the establishment of care plans for individuals with complex care needs, beneficiary self-management assessment and training, and using shared decision-making mechanisms
5. Patient safety and practice assessment, such as through the use of clinical or surgical checklists and practice assessments related to maintaining certification
6. Participation in an alternative payment model

---

[1] Medicare Learning Network, National Provider Call, July 16, 2015, CMS Quality Reporting Programs under the 2016 Medicare Physician Fee Schedule Proposed Rule.

19.6   Tips for Compliance with MIPS

Being prepared is the single most important factor when it comes to incentive-based programs of any sort. First, the financial implications should be thoroughly analyzed and broken down. Every aspect of the potential bonuses or penalties should be understood, and spreadsheets should be developed that ascertain various results and the likelihood of each. Second, the impact on workflow has to be evaluated. This might require testing out some possible scenarios with various clinicians in the practice. Early adopters and champions can be useful, but identifying clinicians who will struggle is also important. One must also make an effort to identify the impact on efficiencies and productivity. An operational and educational action plan is critical to the final phase of preparation. When all of these preparatory steps have occurred, the practice must make a decision. It may be necessary to look at the impact of the changes in years 1, 2, and 3. Sometimes, it makes more sense to continue to prepare internally, but to observe how other practices respond and look for examples of best practices that can be incorporated into your practice.

Preparing the clinicians for these changes is of paramount importance. There are multiple aspects of this that matter. If the practice believes that it will be too costly to implement a program in the first year and thus recognizes that there will be some penalties, warning the clinicians and asking everyone to step it up for a year from a productivity perspective may be necessary. The alternative would be pushing them to implement the program and either working harder or ultimately receiving less pay. Being honest about the situation is always the best policy and increases the likelihood of acceptance of whatever approach the practice decides to take. The changes that need to occur in order for the practice to succeed in these situations require the full buy-in of all of the clinicians and staff.

Staffs are also a critical element in making incentive programs viable. Sometimes the solution will be to utilize medical assistants or clerical staff who are far less expensive than clinicians in order to accomplish the necessary documentation. The staff will also need to be brought along in terms of morale and assuring that everyone in the practice is on the same page.

19.7   Scribes and Cost: Benefit Analysis

The idea of using scribes to help clinicians document their patient visits has evolved with the use of electronic health records. While this may just be a short-term fix on the road to an ultimate long-term solution, it is worth discussing in the context of how to come up with the best approach to addressing programs such as MIPS. The concept of a scribe certainly evolved due to the fact that many clinicians feel uncomfortable documenting in the EHR while seeing a patient.

Clearly, hiring an extra staff person is an expense to the practice. What is the cost of that person? What is the impact on the productivity of the clinician? What is the practical outcome in terms of documenting quality measures? What bonuses might be achieved or what penalties might be avoided? In order to decide on the efficacy of such a program, one must analyze every aspect of the approach. A full cost/benefit analysis should include all of the aspects noted above. Don't assume that using scribes will either save money or lose money. Obtain the necessary data. Do the analysis. Only then can the practice make an informed decision on how to determine the best approach.

Fee for Service: Will It Ever Die?

When we started Senior Care of Colorado in 2001, everyone told us that it was impossible to make a living on a pure fee-for-service Medicare practice. Fortunately, that turned out not to be the case. Today, alternate payment methods such as bundled payments and shared savings are all the rage. So it would seem that it's almost time to forget about fee-for-service. That could not be further from the truth! There are many reasons that having a solid fee-for-service approach built into a practice is important. The first is that it is highly unlikely that the fee-for-service model will go away in our lifetime. This method is so ingrained in our healthcare system that changing it will take decades at best. The other somewhat ironic twist is that even if the government were to do away with fee-for-service tomorrow, most practices, health systems, and insurers would continue to use it because that is what they know!

The fee-for-service model of payment fits neatly into our societies' typical concept of productivity-based service delivery. You get paid for how many widgets that you deliver. There's also the issue of reimbursing someone for the time and effort that they put into delivering a service. In any workplace, there will always be differences in how many hours someone puts in. The question usually is not whether they are working harder, however, but could they work smarter? When you're producing widgets, however, it's the number of widgets produced that matters, unless one person is producing a lower quality of widget. You can begin to see where this is going. We will save the quality discussion for another chapter, but suffice it to say that historically physicians have been paid for delivering a particular service rather than the outcome of that service. Since the outcome is often not known for years, reimbursement for routine care tends to focus on the perceived effort involved in delivering the particular service.

20.1 Healthcare Is a Necessary Commodity

Most people would agree that healthcare is a commodity that everyone ultimately needs. Unfortunately, when you are in need of an acute healthcare service, you generally don't have much choice. Similarly, physicians need to make a living, and

© Springer International Publishing Switzerland 2016
M. Wasserman, *The Business of Geriatrics*, DOI 10.1007/978-3-319-28546-7_20

uncertainty in reimbursement makes it difficult to have a sustainable practice. Hence, a highly predictable payment methodology where a doctor gets paid for an office visit or a procedure in a consistent fashion has become the norm. When the Medicare program was founded, physicians got paid the "usual and customary" fee that they charged. I used to liken it to putting your hand into a pot of gold and pulling out what you thought was a fair amount. This changed with the advent of CPT coding for physicians and DRGs for hospitals.

While we will not go into a lengthy discussion of CPT coding here, suffice it to say that each CPT code represents a widget of sorts. The physician can look at these widgets from a few perspectives. There are time-based methodologies for determining the value of a physician's time. There are also complexity-based approaches related to doctor visits. Finally, there is the payment for a procedure that has been performed. A lot of time and effort has been put into trying to develop a fair system around the CPT coding system. While the fairness of this system is rife with controversy, in general, the system works. In fact, while the system was built primarily for the Medicare program, most commercial insurers use the system as well. Ultimately, each individual practice and practitioner must understand how to account for their productivity so that they will be appropriately reimbursed. All of this occurs within a healthcare system where the patients aren't really involved in this process. One could only imagine the impact of adding a bartering process to occur in real time. On the other hand, for the uninsured, bartering may happen in certain circumstances after the fact, but tends to be based on the fact that the patient can't afford to pay their bill.

Physicians and other clinicians want to be able to have a steady income or salary, so uncertainty in reimbursement methodologies is anathema to the practicing physician. Hence, even in health systems that receive capitated payments, physicians generally receive a salary and may receive productivity-based bonuses. With the advent of managed care over the past 30 years, there are circumstances where physicians earn bonuses based on cost savings or adoption of quality measures. The "new" Medicare shared savings model assures that this concept will continue into the future. With that said, will fee-for-service ever die?

20.2 Change Usually Occurs Slowly

While the penetration of managed care has risen, and while the government has essentially mandated a future of alternative payment methodologies, change still occurs slowly. There are still a lot of markets where fee-for-service is still the norm. In these markets, it is paramount that a practice recognizes and understands the working of the fee-for-service model. In fact, there are actually opportunities to leverage fee-for-service with alternative payment models to maximize the value of both. At the same time, there are potential potholes and pitfalls in delivering care while receiving different types of reimbursement.

Getting clinicians to shift from a productivity-based mentality will be difficult enough, but getting large practices and health systems to make the change will have to occur slowly. As we have stated in other chapters, even if a clinician is providing excellent quality of care, the absolute productivity of that clinician is important insofar as the need to determine the number of clinicians to care for all of the patients in a practice. For example, if 60 patients need to be seen in a day, a balance needs to be achieved that allows for the delivery of quality care. At the same time, the overhead and salaries needed to provide the care cannot exceed the revenue that is received.

20.3 Focus on Quality

As both a physician and geriatrician alike, we have taken an oath to care for our patients. I strongly believe that most physicians take this oath seriously. Knowingly providing a service that is known to be harmful, or of no value, would be unethical. The major issue in the geriatric realm is that we have very limited data relating to evidence-based care. Most physicians practice based on what they were taught in medical school and residency and truly don't know any better. At the same time, the history of medical care is rife with stories of traditional treatments that are ultimately proven to be ineffective. Nevertheless, most every physician would like to think that they are practicing with the patient's interest in mind. Most clinicians would state that they are focused on providing a high quality of care. The reader is reminded of our basic premise that a geriatric medical approach to care is the path to quality care. Because, at this point in time, that approach also tends to be cost-effective is quite fortuitous.

To many people, especially everyone who dissuaded Dr. Murphy and myself from founding Senior Care of Colorado in 2001, the geriatric medical approach to care was not a profitable one in a fee-for-service environment. *We did not accept this premise.* Similar to many other business models, we felt that providing a quality service must ultimately be profitable. Traditional supply and demand principles would assure this to be the case. To this day, I will hold to the belief that this must be true, or the healthcare system will ultimately fail. If one is to believe this premise, it becomes necessary to fit the widgets into the necessary holes.

If there is one thing that is true about delivering a quality geriatric product, it is that one will have no shortage of patients! This is an important concept for many reasons, which we will address in short order. First, however, I must share a story. It was soon after we founded Senior Care of Colorado that my staff told me the story of an older gentleman who came into our office and asked if we accepted Medicare. When he was told that we did, he burst into tears! It turned out that we were the eighth office that he had gone to, and we were the first practice that told him that we would care for him. This is actually not an unusual occurrence. Many years ago, I was told by a primary care physician that the maximum percentage of Medicare patients a practice should accept was 20 %. This was the prevailing wisdom at the time and actually continues to be so in many markets. Of interest, the government believes that there is adequate access to care for Medicare beneficiaries, but this data is primarily based on information that includes the availability of specialists.

As we live in a world with a diminishing number of primary care physicians, and a growing number of older adults, the problem of finding a primary care doctor will continue to grow.

20.4   Leveraging Patients Along the Continuum

As we have seen in the pages of this book, *geriatricians are needed everywhere along the continuum of care.* This creates opportunities to leverage the fact that we are a magnet for older adult patients. Senior Care of Colorado was a living, breathing example of this. As soon as we "opened our doors," we were in high demand. We never advertised, primarily out of fear of overwhelming ourselves. Aside from the fact that we were never in need of additional clinic patients, we were immediately sought out by nursing homes and assisted living facilities. The reason for this is fairly obvious. Our outpatient population were "feeders" for higher levels of care along the continuum. There was a perception, right or wrong, that we might supply residents for assisted living facilities and nursing homes alike. As one has read in an earlier chapter, this perception actually contributed to our being investigated by the OIG. Nevertheless, business is business, and perceptions can be utilized if managed properly.

There was no question that as geriatricians we had expertise in the care of the frail elderly. Considering the fact that, at the time we started Senior Care of Colorado, there were still nursing home doctors who were retired surgeons and pediatricians, we had something to offer to the community. We approached nursing facilities and let it be known that we were interested in attending to their patient population. In addition to welcoming us as clinicians, we were also inundated by requests to provide medical direction. While facilities made these offers out of the perception that patients might follow along, we accepted out of our desire to *improve the quality of care in their facilities.*

In order to effectively leverage ones position, the service must match up with the opportunity. Nursing homes can be a challenging place to work. Phone calls, both day and night, have been known to overwhelm the resources of many practices. We quickly realized that providing more on-site care was the key to reducing phone calls, increasing revenue, and reducing expenses. In fact, having clinicians on-site most days of the week became its own marketing approach. This leads to continued growth of our practice, which ultimately took on a life of its own.

The move into assisted living facilities was a natural outgrowth of this process, which has been described in a previous chapter. Nevertheless, similar to our nursing home situation, our assisted living population led to their own leverage points. Clearly, if our clinic patients were perceived as being "valuable" to nursing facilities, the assisted living patients were of even greater value. That value took on another level of importance when it came to the insurance companies.

20.5   Leveraging Care Along the Continuum

Insurance companies definitely took note of our practice for a multitude of reasons. Over the past 40 years, there has been an increasing emphasis on moving Medicare patients into HMOs and Medicare Advantage programs. Those programs all have marketing departments. They desire to add more patients to their programs. Our practice focused on fee-for-service patients. We were a potential "feeder" for Medicare Advantage programs. As we have recounted earlier, when our practice was owned and managed by GeriMed of America, we had made a dedicated attempt to enlist all of our patients into the local HMO. The outcome of this was quite mixed and we still had a preponderance of pure fee-for-service patients. As Medigap insurance costs grew, and Medicare Advantage programs offered lower premium products, there was an incentive for patients to join such programs.

This became a "perfect storm" for us to both convert existing patients and market to patients in the community. Ultimately, we developed shared savings arrangements with the local Medicare Advantage program which would bring us additional revenue. Furthermore, our existence along the rest of the continuum brought additional opportunities. Our ability to provide daily care in many skilled nursing homes was appealing to the insurance companies, as was our approach to care that encouraged discharging patients home as soon as possible. As I have previously recounted our experience negotiating a much higher reimbursement rate, we definitely had the ability to leverage our position. Of course, leveraging too much can backfire. In the long run, however, our position in the community led to excellent relationships with the Medicare Advantage programs.

20.6   A Missed Opportunity

When GeriMed developed our full-risk program in Florida, we stubbornly held to the idea that fee-for-service was not profitable and thus focused primarily on managed care patients. This extended from the office into the nursing homes, where we were definitely able to leverage our managed care clinic population into relationships with the local nursing facilities. There was no question that they saw our practice as an opportunity to have additional patients admitted. We could even directly admit residents and bypass the hospital, which they definitely loved. This also created a win-win situation for us to develop such programs with a willing partner who perceived potential benefit. The opportunity that we missed on was that we held to our stubborn belief that fee-for-service care was not the way to go and thus missed out on a huge opportunity to literally corner the nursing home market in Central Florida.

A geriatric practice should always be on the lookout for opportunities to leverage their patient base along the continuum. Whether the patients are fee-for-service or belong to a Medicare Advantage plan should be of no consequence. In fact, *having a mix of patients actually provides a great opportunity to demonstrate ones commitment to high quality of care!* I'll never forget having a patient's daughter get upset with me for not wanting to admit her father to the hospital. She accused me of making my decision based on potential monetary gain. The irony was that the patient was a fee-for-service patient! The monetary gain would have actually been in admitting the patient to the hospital at the time.

20.7   Demonstrating the Quality Commitment

A consistent commitment to the geriatric approach to care regardless of payor source is a huge opportunity for a practice to insulate itself from accusations that it is making treatment decisions based on monetary gain. In the fee-for-service environment, keeping patients out of the hospital or not performing expensive procedures is clearly not in the pure financial interest of the practice, while in the managed care setting can provide for lucrative bonuses. As we opened this chapter, however, we noted the core belief that physicians truly want to focus on providing the highest quality of care for their patients.

Ironically, it has been my experience that geriatricians and other geriatric healthcare professionals are often leery of clinical decisions that make money. Hence, if they are unsure of whether to hospitalize a patient or not, they might choose to put the patient in the hospital to avoid any perception that they are trying to make or save money by avoiding the hospitalization. This is why a geriatric practice must put energy into constantly educating their providers on the value of the geriatric approach to care. Practicing a consistent approach regardless of payor source is a very profound way of reinforcing this message.

20.8   Leverage, Leverage, Leverage

The continued focus in this chapter on leverage is at the heart of why a practice needs to continue to embrace the importance of understanding fee-for-service reimbursement. Ignoring any percentage of a market limits ones effectiveness in maximizing all of the available opportunities. By either ignoring or avoiding fee-for-service opportunities, practices will inherently limit themselves. Additionally, there are many times that one can leverage their fee-for-service population with their managed care population. *Finally, leveraging the perception of the value of the geriatric approach to care across all care approaches and settings is an opportunity that should not be missed!*

Competition: Not an Effective Strategy

21

One of the fascinating things that I've seen in the geriatric marketplace is the tendency for practices to compete with one another in communities where there is actually a paucity of experienced providers. Perhaps it's human nature that invites competition, but while two practices are fighting it out trying to get patients in one facility, there is another facility nearby that is lacking in effective coverage. No one wins in this situation. In fact, everyone loses, including the patients. Furthermore, whereas competition may invite innovation and efficiencies in some businesses, in geriatrics it tends to reduce efficiencies and adds overhead. One of the reasons for that is that the laws of supply and demand have essentially been suspended when it comes to the practice of geriatrics. We have a huge demand and a poor supply of geriatricians. We also have a complex array of circumstances that interfere with traditional market-based concepts.

21.1 It's Personal, Not Business

Being competitive is human nature, and there is a natural tendency to want to keep up with your competitors. We had some situations a number of years ago in Denver with a variety of former employees who decided that they were going to compete with our practice in the nursing home market. Keep in mind that there are a lot of nursing homes in the Denver metropolitan area, and only so many geriatricians. We were initially surprised to find a former colleague enter nursing facilities where we were the predominant provider. Ironically, it rarely turned out well for the other clinician. Breaking into a nursing facility generally means that you have very few patients, which means you are running around town from facility to facility with low efficiencies. On the other hand, entering a facility that has trouble finding doctors and offering your services can quickly lead to a large volume of patients.

Why do individuals do this? The main answer seems to be that it's personal, not business. It should be obvious that this is the wrong approach. *Business decisions should be based on logistics and facts, not emotion.* In many of the cases that I am

© Springer International Publishing Switzerland 2016
M. Wasserman, *The Business of Geriatrics*, DOI 10.1007/978-3-319-28546-7_21

alluding to, it was clear that the former employee felt that they had something to prove by trying to compete with us on our own turf. The problem for them should be obvious. We had the home court advantage. We had relationships, we had efficiencies already developed. While there are customer acquisition costs in any business, those costs can be quite high when trying to build a nursing home practice in a building that already has adequate coverage.

21.2   Don't React Emotionally

It truly is business and not personal. That needs to be the key response when another person or business invades ones territory. Reacting emotionally, lashing out, and fighting back in any way are the wrong approaches. Over time, we learned that the best response was to focus on what we did the best, providing high-quality care and a high level of customer service. In fact, there was one situation where the "invading" practice actually managed to initially secure the bulk of the admissions (perhaps they brought better doughnuts to the nurses). Over time, they were unable to provide the same level of service that we had been providing for some time, and ultimately the bulk of the business came back to us. Being patient not only paid off on a practical level, but allowed us to be perceived positively by the facility staff and administration. I remember that our clinicians at this facility were very upset and wanted us to "do something." That would have been the wrong approach.

As we have discussed in an earlier chapter, it is not unusual for a nursing home to bring new physicians into their building in the hopes of securing more admissions. The irony of this approach is that it rarely works. Nevertheless, I've seen it happen many times. This is one of the examples of how market forces can be skewed in the long-term care arena. In most other industries, if you have a reliable vendor delivering excellent and consistent services, why would you want to purposely bring in competition? The answer clearly has to do with a facility's perception that the new physician will bring additional patients. On the other hand, it ignores other important variables in the equation that relate to the quality of the actual service being delivered. While being on the receiving end of this competitive challenge can be difficult, taking the high road is generally the best response. The nursing staff knows who responds to their phone calls the fastest!

21.3   The Demographic Imperative

There is no question that the baby boom is unlike anything our society has ever seen. The segment of the population that is over the age of 65 is growing faster than any other age category. The opportunities for a geriatric practice are boundless under these circumstances. The fact that the United States has a paucity of geriatricians heightens the potential opportunities even more. Despite a push to maintain frail older adults in their homes, the growth in the population will assure a significant number of residents in nursing facilities. The assisted living industry continues to expand, and there is probably no end in sight to this growth. A cottage industry of group homes, each housing six people, ensures a steady supply of patients for geriatricians. Finally, the reemergence of house calls provides yet another opportunity for geriatric clinicians.

The historical approach by primary care physicians to minimize the percentage of Medicare beneficiaries in their practice to under 20 % creates clear opportunities in the outpatient setting. Unfortunately, from a societal perspective, this has not been a setting that geriatricians have flocked to. Furthermore, the profit margin in this setting is still fairly narrow. For these reasons, this arena will continue to offer a wide open chance to deliver geriatric care. Nursing homes present another, more variable and complex, story.

21.4 The Financial Lure of Nursing Homes

The fact is that nursing homes have plenty of residents, no waiting room, and a population that has very little choice as to who their doctor is. I have seen retired pediatricians and surgeons develop large nursing home practices. While some of them gravitate well to a geriatric approach to care, that is not always the case. The financial reality is that one can see a lot of patients in one day in a facility. Suffice it to say that occasionally human nature may trump the Hippocratic Oath.

Into this professional void comes opportunities for geriatricians to shine. Knowledge of the frail elderly as well as the inner workings of nursing facilities puts geriatricians in position to take advantage of their skill set. *A geriatric practice can benefit from the obvious difference in their approach to care by highlighting the elements that make them both the right clinicians and the right partners.* In today's healthcare world, skilled nursing facilities understand the value of a geriatric practice that is well connected with the community and the entire continuum of care.

On the other hand, in communities that have large number of geriatricians, the competition in nursing facilities can be quite intense. Practitioners know that this is the most lucrative setting to practice in, and it isn't uncommon to find many physicians vying for medical director positions and the opportunity to care for residents. It is important to do ones homework in such situations. Even in communities with a significant number of geriatric clinicians, there still tends to be many facilities that do not have adequate coverage. Some of the reasons might involve the perceived quality of such facilities.

Instead of steering away from the less popular nursing facilities, a geriatric practice should see a significant opportunity. The chance to become a medical director and guide a nursing home to continuous improvement is one approach that a practice can take. On the other hand, just providing daily visits and being responsive to phone calls can quickly lead to caring for the majority of residents in a facility. With that said, nursing homes aren't the only opportunity along the continuum, and in a competitive market, a practice should seek out the patients who don't have the most access to physicians. Assisted living facilities (ALFs) are definitely that place.

21.5   Assisted Living Facilities and Willie Sutton

Willie Sutton was the famous bank robber who, when asked why he robbed banks, said "that's where the money is." *Assisted living facilities are definitely where the frail older population resides.* Historically, they were not deemed to be the best place for a geriatric practice to flourish. As we have noted in an earlier chapter, that has changed. First of all, the reimbursement is quite adequate and if economies of scale are fully utilized, this is a great opportunity! While there is a tendency for most practices to look first at nursing facilities, if one is in a competitive environment, they should definitely cast their eyes on the local assisted living facilities.

Growing an assisted living practice takes more effort than a nursing home practice, but the results can be very positive. Additionally, it is not uncommon for assisted living residents to ultimately require nursing home care. Thus, by building an assisted living practice, one is also building toward their nursing home practice as well. The work it takes to grow an assisted living practice entails paying attention to the staff at the facility and learning the ins and outs of whatever systems they have in place.

Competition within an assisted living facility is less frequent, especially due to the logistics needed to have an effective practice in a facility. Furthermore, unless a practice is incredibly large, it is unlikely that it can manage to care for residents in a lot of nursing homes and assisted living facilities. It can also be more difficult to set up an effective system of care within an assisted living facility. On the other hand, a practice that pays attention to structure, process, and workflow can position themselves very effectively in an ALF.

21.6   Marketing Matters

It is always remarkable how many physicians can still be rude to the staff in nursing facilities. In order to avoid being susceptible to competition, it really behooves individual clinicians and a geriatric practice to follow basic marketing principles. Letting staff know how much they are appreciated goes a long way. These are people who work very hard, often in lower paying jobs. They are not perfect, and they will make mistakes. I'll never forget getting a 3 a.m. phone call from a nursing home nurse many years ago. She called to give me a normal lab value! I instinctively yelled at her. Laying in bed, feeling bad about having yelled at a nurse, I called her back and apologized. From that day forward, if a nurse called me for a nonsensical reason, I took the opportunity to educate the nurse.

Having a system in place that improves the communication between the practice and the facility goes a long way. We had a building where we had clinicians available 5 days a week and over 8 h a day. That building was responsible for the highest number of phone calls to our triage system! It made no sense. Ultimately, we worked to develop a system on each unit that improved the communication between our clinicians and the nursing staff. While this might appear to be more of an operational issue, in fact, it has a significant marketing impact. Nurses don't like being interrupted by a call back from a physician any more than the physician likes to be interrupted by a call. We're all in this together!

21.7 Sell Your Expertise!

In the midst of the demographic imperative that the baby boom has brought us, geriatricians are a very limited commodity. While it continues to frustrate many of us, governmental solutions to Medicare's growing financial challenges almost never include the words geriatrician or geriatric medicine. The fact that we often take our own skills for granted does not help us. *Throughout the pages of this book, we have outlined a variety of areas in which geriatricians and geriatric practices can have a positive influence on both quality and healthcare costs.* The geriatric approach to care can be the linchpin for this positive influence!

I once had a meeting with a congressional staffer, who lamented that geriatricians were generally too passive in their approach to presenting their expertise. On the other hand, the interventional cardiologists would pound their fists on the table and talk about how many lives they saved! The irony of this relates back to something that I learned early in my career. Physicians trained by a traditional medical education system tend to believe that they have to intervene. Geriatricians are often looked at askance for taking more holistic and nontraditional approaches. Too many of us have bought into this and are not forceful enough in advocating for what we do.

If you are a geriatrician, a geriatric nurse practitioner, a geriatric physicians' assistant, or a geriatric nurse specialist, you believe in what you do. You understand the risks of polypharmacy. You try very hard to keep your patients out of an acute hospital. You focus on quality of life and function. You are also passionate about the geriatric approach to care. *Let some of that passion come out when you are promoting what you do!* Don't be afraid to share examples of what works and what doesn't work. Just because there are not a lot of studies demonstrating the best approach to caring for frail 95-year-old women doesn't mean that our collective experience has no value.

21.8 The "n"'s the Thing

Many years ago I did some speaking about cholinesterase inhibitors, still the main line of medications for treating Alzheimer's disease. This was actually one of the few drugs where studies had been performed in older adults. When looking at some of the clinical trials, it became obvious to me that many of these trials had "n"'s of less than a few hundred subjects. Our practice often saw more than that many people with Alzheimer's disease in a single day! It became clear to me that while geriatricians may not have the luxury of evidence-based literature to support their approach to care, what we had was experience. For this reason, I have often asked my fellow clinicians about their approaches to care of many common geriatric syndromes.

This has allowed me to augment my body of experience and to transcend the non-existent clinical trials. Does this represent a rigid scientific process? No. Is it more evidence than most specialists have for the procedures they perform or the medications that they give to frail older adults? Absolutely!

It is important for us to take our knowledge and experience and to promote what we do. The market forces are often aligned against us. While hospitals now have incentives to reduce readmissions, they still want to keep their beds full. Specialists get paid more (at this time) for doing expensive procedures. Some of the new alternate payment models will try to change this, but it won't take long for the health systems to realize that they are paying their specialists a lot to do less. There will be push back! We have to be prepared to stand up and vouch for our approach. We have to use whatever available literature we have. We have to dig deep into our body of knowledge and experience and promote the geriatric approach to care. *At the end of the day, it is about delivering quality care and providing excellent customer service. It's not about thinking competitively.*

Getting the Most Out of Providers

22

This chapter is about the Holy Grail of healthcare management. Physicians, in particular, seem to be the most challenging employees to manage. Their training leads them to think of themselves as both the leader and decision-maker. Following direction from others can therefore be a difficult proposition. Confounding this is the fact that the nuances of coding seem far more difficult to learn than treating congestive heart failure or diabetes. We have also discussed the fact that geriatricians want to focus on caring for their patients and see any time and energy that is spent focused on coding and billing to be a distraction.

In an earlier chapter, we talked about the psychology of geriatricians. I have encountered many geriatric clinicians who don't want to feel as if they are making money off their patients. While this is clearly a challenge, it is still possible to get geriatricians to be productive. In fact, clinicians who work in geriatrics are among some of the hardest working and most dedicated people that I have had the privilege of working with. It would not be surprising to find that many geriatricians feel more comfortable in a salaried environment. Unfortunately, even in this type of reimbursement schema, they must still ultimately be responsible for their productivity. Hence, the rub. How does one approach this complex issue?

22.1 Patient Care Is the Key

We came face-to-face with this issue at Senior Care of Colorado after a particularly rough year. In order to assure the long-term success of the practice, we really had to focus on every provider's productivity. We had developed a system that was working, but was negatively impacting morale. Our revenue had increased, but we realized that we had to do something or risk losing some very good clinicians. We came up with a partial solution. They were called patient care units, or PCUs. *By focusing on recognizing the fact that clinicians were getting credit for the care they provided, we changed the conversation.* It seems simple, but it worked. The concept of PCUs was predicated on developing an administrative "cross-walk" between the units and

© Springer International Publishing Switzerland 2016
M. Wasserman, *The Business of Geriatrics*, DOI 10.1007/978-3-319-28546-7_22

the revenue that those units ultimately represented. We did not share that connection with the clinicians. As silly as it sounds, this method worked pretty well! It also helped us to explain to our clinicians the value of the time that they spent caring for their complex patients.

Geriatricians want to deliver quality care to their patients. They want to be able to practice a brand of medicine that is generally not favored in many practice environments. Supporting the geriatric approach to care can lend itself to a significant increase in the morale of the clinician, which makes some of the other educational tasks that we will cover easier to accept. *It is critical that the clinicians in a geriatrics practice feel that their primary mission is to care for their patients!*

22.2 Valuing What One Does

It's always been remarkable to see how geriatricians tend to minimize the complexity and value of what they do. Caring for the most frail of all patients in the healthcare system is not an easy task. One can liken the work of geriatricians to that of chess grandmasters. Chess grandmasters are not good at what they do because they have a better memory or can see more moves ahead. They are good because they are pattern thinkers and can view the complex chess board with a clarity that others can't. Being a geriatrician is very similar. If one focused solely on each individual disease, every patient visit could take hours, and there is no guarantee that the physician would have any grasp of how to manage that patient. Geriatricians must incorporate highly complex medical information into the psychosocial aspects of a patient's life. They also have to do this without much, if any, evidence-based literature. So, why do geriatricians minimize the value and complexity of what they do?

In a previous chapter, I outlined some of the issues that plague geriatric healthcare providers in relation to their psychological makeup. This may be one of the most important elements involved in getting the most out of those providers. I can't begin to relate the number of times that I have asked geriatricians how often they have coded the highest level of office visit codes. The response of "almost never" does not correspond with my next question, "how often do you spend more than 40 min with a patient?" If a clinician spends 40 min with a patient and spends more than 50 % of that time in education and counseling (almost a given under those circumstances), they have the precise criteria necessary for coding the highest level code. Why don't they? First of all, it seems that they often don't feel like they deserve to bill the higher code!

Having a geriatrician leader who reinforces the value of the geriatric approach to care is a very important aspect of a successful geriatric practice. Since geriatricians often minimize the value of their care, it is necessary to regularly reinforce that value. While one of the reasons for undervaluing their worth has to do with their perception of the monetary aspects of coding and billing, there is also a tendency to undervalue the actual effort that they put in. Too many geriatricians have burned out by not recognizing the intensity of the work necessary to care for complex frail elderly. *One of the core missions of a geriatric practice is to assure that every clinician fully understands the value of the care they deliver!*

22.3   Code for the Work that Is Performed

The single most important coding item to educate clinicians on is that they must code for the actual work that they do! I can't count the number of times that I have had a geriatrician, nurse practitioner, or physician assistant tell me that they put in a 12 h/day, only to have their coding correspond to under 4 h! While there are a multitude of reasons for this behavior, we have reviewed those reasons throughout this book. So, what does a practice do? *The greatest tool that one can utilize to get clinicians to code properly is a daily diary* that is reviewed and correlated to their concomitant coding for that period of time.

In order to affect the coding behavior of a geriatrician, it is necessary to maintain an ongoing educational process. It is also necessary to monitor their coding behavior in order to identify changes that require updating that education. When changes in coding patterns are seen, utilizing a two-day diary and then following that up with a face-to-face meeting can be very powerful. The practice also has to have its ear to the ground in regard to rumors or concerns that the government is targeting or auditing the practice. The fear of such audits often works as a counterbalance to all of the educational efforts that a practice undertakes.

Assuring that clinicians accurately code for work that is appropriately performed is the single most important focus of a geriatric practice. Ignoring this issue is one of the most dangerous things a practice can do. There is actually a second angle to this focus, which is monitoring for overcoding. There is always the occasional clinician who flaunts the coding rules and code levels that are higher than the actual work performed. Needless to say, a geriatric practice must be diligent in monitoring for this type of behavior and must act quickly in response to such coding. It is also necessary for the practice to recode and re-bill the overcoded visits and to document the education given to the clinician in their personnel record. All the while, the practice must take great pains not to create fear in other clinicians in regard to coding practices!

22.4   Managing Clinicians Is Worth the Effort

One of the interesting administrative battles we used to have in our practice was valuing the time necessary for a geriatrician manager to oversee the coding practices of the geriatricians, nurse practitioners, and physician assistants in the practice. It is critical to recognize that undercoding by just one level can often lead to a 30 % loss of revenue. Clinician's who are not coding appropriately can easily cost a practice 10–20 % in lost revenue in a heartbeat! *The time spent by a geriatrician leader to oversee the productivity and coding habits of the other clinicians can be the most cost-effective decision that a practice takes.* Do the math, and you'll have the answer!

Since many clinicians will spend a significant amount of time in the field, it is often necessary for the geriatrician leader to spend a half-day out in the field with them. Many nursing homes and assisted living facilities have their own challenges and oftentimes such an experience will highlight operational issues that may be impacting a clinician's productivity. One also cannot overestimate the value of a clinician seeing the interest that their leader has in assuring that they fully understand what is going on "in the trenches."

22.5 Marketing Is Not a Bad Word

As I have recounted elsewhere in this book, *I often tell my new patients that if they want a doctor who will order lots of tests, put them on lots of medications, send them to lots of specialists, and admit them to the hospital at the drop of a hat, then I am not their guy.* First of all, I am telling my patients the truth. That is who I am as a geriatrician. I am passionate about delivering the highest quality of care to older adults, and I care deeply about doing so. Secondly, I am actually marketing myself! To many physicians, the idea of marketing oneself is anathema. What they often don't realize is that marketing is also about relationship building. And building a relationship with one's patients improves the ability to communicate and care for that person.

Geriatric practices are highly sensitive to the continuum of care. Skilled nursing admissions may represent a significant source of revenue to a practice. Adding more residents of a group home or assisted living facility can increase the efficiency and therefore productivity of a clinician. Some component of time spent in the field should be focused on representing the value that the practice brings to that facility. This is also marketing, but again, it is relationship building. Complementing the nurses and CNAs in a nursing home will not only strengthen the relationship with that facility but will improve the communication that occurs between the facility staff and the clinician. That level of communication can lead to improved care as clinicians are notified earlier and more effectively about changes in condition of residents.

As the geriatrician leaves a nursing facility at the end of the day, it is inevitable that they run into the family member of a resident. That person may want to ask a question of the clinician. It may be that the clinician has already seen the resident, or perhaps they haven't. Instead of viewing this circumstance as a nuisance, it must be viewed as an opportunity. First, it's an opportunity to improve the care of the patient, as it is possible that the information received has not previously been communicated. Second, it's an incredible marketing opportunity! Family members of residents in nursing and assisted living facilities alike are not used to communicating with the doctor. These are golden opportunities. As an additional note, if the patient had not been seen that day, the clinician should definitely consider going back to briefly see the resident so that they can write a note and bill for the work that they did in addressing the issue that the family member had. The key to this is to document that "the patient was seen at the request of his daughter regarding…"

22.6 Physicians Are People Too

As physicians are typically very independent minded and self-sufficient, it is not unusual for a practice to ignore the need to coddle them to some degree. First of all, *listen to any complaints that your clinicians have!* One doesn't have to react to each and every complaint, but it is critical to listen to each one and to get back to the clinician in a timely fashion with some feedback. The feedback doesn't even have to be a solution, as often there is not one. In those cases, an explanation will go a long way.

Physicians are not immune to having psychological issues such as depression. They may also be prone to substance abuse. It is remarkable how easy it is for a practice and for others along the continuum of care to enable such physicians. Getting the most out of your clinicians means paying attention to them as individuals. Are they happy? Have you been getting complaints from patients? Have nursing facilities been complaining? *An annual evaluation should be done at a minimum, and it's often useful to meet the clinician in the field so that you are not having a significant impact on their time.*

22.7   Monitor Fair Market Value

Like any business and any employee, one should pay attention to what the market value of your clinicians are. The last thing you want to do is to lose a good clinician because they can make a few thousand more dollars a year with a competitor. With that said, it's not always just about money. Your clinicians want to be appreciated and they want to know that you listen and pay attention to them. You don't always have to do everything that they want. In fact, it may be more beneficial to take the time to explain why you can't give them an increase. For example, pointing out some of the nonmonetary benefits of the practice such as more reasonable call can accomplish more than just saying that you can't afford to give them an increase.

At the same time, if the practice is doing well and you can assure that your clinicians are being paid at fair market value, you should not hesitate to do so. Losing a clinician is one of the most costly hits a practice can take. It ultimately costs between 100 and 200,000 dollars to replace a physician, and over half that amount to replace a nurse practitioner or physician assistant. Those costs include recruitment costs, but more importantly, the time it takes to get a new clinician up to speed on appropriate coding and the workflow of the practice itself. It not only pays to get the most out of your clinicians, but to retain them as well!

22.8   Healthcare Is a Business, Not a Commodity

This is ultimately the greatest challenge that healthcare faces, and medical practices are not immune to this. As I said at the outset of this book, the credo of "no margin, no mission" still holds true. At the same time, for geriatricians and a geriatric practice, the mission must also be adhered to. One can do both, as our experience at both GeriMed of America and Senior Care of Colorado can attest to. At the core of delivering on the geriatric mission are the clinicians. Without clinicians who are trained, passionate, and dedicated to the geriatric approach to care, the geriatric model of care will not work. On one level, we must cater to our clinicians, but on another level, we must hold them accountable. That is the tightrope that we walk, but it is a walk worth taking.

Electronic Health Records

23

Electronic health records (EHRs) have become the new solution to everything in healthcare. Whether that is true or not doesn't really matter. What does matter is that EHRs are here to stay and we have to deal with that fact for many reasons. The first reason is simple. Those that don't use an EHR will be penalized. The second reason is more complex. EHRs have the "potential" to improve efficiencies and even improve the delivery of care. But there are multiple reasons that I say they have the "potential" to do this. In fact, the ultimate success of a medical practice may revolve around this single issue.

I think that some background would be useful in trying to help the reader understand the myriad issues that stem from a discussion of electronic records. I grew up in a world before personal computers. However, I was among the first to own one once I started practicing. While I am in no way tech savvy, I happen to be an excellent typist. This has been an important requirement for those who try to utilize EHRs. When I joined GeriMed of America in 1994, they were beginning to develop computer software to assist in the care coordination process. Four years later, we had developed software that allowed us to place computers in every one of our exam rooms. We were on the leading edge of this movement and in some ways on the "bleeding edge."

23.1 Avoid the Bleeding Edge

Taking a measured approach to develop an electronic health record system is a critical component toward being successful. One has to stay away from the glitz and glitter of expensive systems that do more than is necessary. It is also important that the system be very friendly to the likes of physicians, nurse practitioners, physician assistants, medical assistants, and receptionists alike. Problems with anyone of these members of the team will create inefficiencies. I have always had a simple rule. If an EHR adds a single second to the day of a clinician, it will be a problem. While this may not be entirely accurate, it is an excellent starting point for making decisions regarding adopting EHR technology.

© Springer International Publishing Switzerland 2016
M. Wasserman, *The Business of Geriatrics*, DOI 10.1007/978-3-319-28546-7_23

23.1.1 EHRs and Workflow

One of the catch 22s of EHRs today is that they are "billing centric." This chapter will not be a treatise on the ideal EHR. From a quality of care perspective, future EHRs must become patient care centric. However, that is unlikely to happen anytime soon. In the meantime, it is critical that EHRs capture the critical data that is necessary for the financial success of a practice. First and foremost, this means billing. An EHR must be friendly to the coding and billing process. The next area that is coming to the fore is the ability of an EHR to capture an ongoing and changing array of required metrics. Most of these metrics have been defined as "quality measures," and while that definition may be debatable at times, once again, it is what we have to deal with. Today's EHRs must be able to effectively and efficiently capture the required metrics. Finally, an EHR must be able to be melded into the workflow of a practice. This is often the most overlooked aspect of EHRs. The software is often developed in the dark room of a computer programmer hunched over their computer.

I was fortunate at GeriMed to have the services of a certifiable computer programming genius by the name of Doug Selzler. Doug used a programing software called Clarion™ that allowed him to do what seemed to be the work of many people. Around the time, I had also read an article that stated that the more programmers you had, the slower the development process would be. I'm not an expert on the subject, but Doug built a workable EHR by himself. But, he had help! The help was from the clinicians and staff that worked in my office. Doug would come into the office and observe how the system was working. I would even bring him into the exam room with me (with the patient's approval), so that we could tweak the system as I saw my patients. Ironically, one of the biggest mistakes I made was teaming him up with a clinician who was "into" computers. They spoke the same language, which was the problem. In fact, I generally saw my role as being a translator for him. It is imperative that both clinicians and staff are able to communicate the necessary requirements for an EHR to be friendly to the daily workflow. One of the problems with many of today's EHRs is that they can't be tweaked by individual practices. This makes it more difficult to align the EHR with the day-to-day operations of the practice. However, it doesn't make it impossible!

23.2 Making a Choice

When I resigned my position as President of GeriMed and co-founded Senior Care of Colorado, we actually continued to use GeriMed's EHR for awhile. The problem was that I was now running a private practice and did not have the capital or wherewithal to continue to fund software development for a product that wasn't even my own. Ultimately, we went out and bought another EHR. There were things it did, especially from a coding and billing perspective that far exceeded GeriMed's system. On the other hand, from a care coordination and clinical geriatric perspective, it was lacking. That said, we had to work with it. When you can't change your EHR to match your workflow, you have to adjust your workflow to match your EHR. We evaluated office functionality from the point of the patient coming to the front desk to the time they left the office. This takes time and energy that most offices don't believe they have. However, they cannot afford not to spend the time!

What were the advantages of having an EHR in the exam room? For those of us who could type well, especially without looking at the keyboard, this was a no brainer! I could see my patient, type my note, and be out of the exam room and on to the next patient. My documentation was complete, my billing was done, and I had no extra work to do at the end of the day. That was me. On the other hand, we had other clinicians that couldn't type; they would keep notes and type in their documentation at the end of the day. This was horrible, to say the least. Over time, we worked on simplifying templates and procedures in order to make the documentation easier for even the poorest of typists. We encouraged time-based billing, but that still presented a problem for poor typists insofar as they had problems documenting what they did during the visit.

23.3   Develop a Mantra

We ultimately developed a mantra. That mantra was that a clinician needed to complete their note before they left the exam room. We backed it up with the reality that writing a note later in the day was wrong on multiple levels. First, one had to remember everything that they did. Secondly, by finishing the note while seeing the patient, the clinician was able to leave the patient with instructions and plans. If they made additional decisions while completing a note late in the day, they would have to call the patient (which is uncompensated). Honestly, there was always somewhat of a bell-shaped curve when it comes to how our clinicians responded to this approach. Ultimately, some of them just sucked it up and put in the extra work at the end of the day. I was always concerned that this would lead to burnout in those providers, which in fact happened to many of them. There were also clinicians who focused so much on the computer that patients weren't happy. Their documentation was excellent, and they were efficient, but patient satisfaction wasn't ideal. We tried to encourage these clinicians to at least tell the patient that they were using the EHR for the betterment of their overall health and to apologize for looking at the computer rather than the patient. This actually worked to some degree, although recent literature suggests that this is an important issue that is simmering beneath the surface in regard to the value of EHRs.

As I noted, coding and billing are arguably the most important aspects of an EHR when it comes to financial success. It's actually important to break down the two components. From the perspective of the clinician, not only is it critical that they be trained to understand the coding rules, it is important that they understand it in the context of the particular EHR that they are using. Some EHRs actually have "smarts" that help the clinician determine the appropriate code. On the other hand, it is incumbent upon the practice to know if those "smarts" are accurate. It is probably not hard to imagine that most existing EHRs have been built with a conservative view of billing. If the EHR leads to clinicians undercoding, that will not be a good thing. At the same time, one must monitor the use of an EHR by the same clinicians, as there might be opportunities to "cut and paste" in ways that will enhance the coding, but might run afoul of the regulations. While I'd like to believe that this isn't true, it is also possible for the same "cut and paste" approach to lead clinicians to document for work they haven't done.

23.4   Beware of Overcoding

Similarly, EHRs may encourage overcoding, although that is not solely in the domain of the responsibility of an EHR. The desire to make more money in a productivity-driven system can test the ethics of any clinician. EHRs may at times make this easier to do. At the same time, the documentation requirements of an EHR makes it possible to more easily monitor the coding patterns of clinicians. *It is important for the practice to develop internal metrics by which to monitor clinician coding patterns.*

The opportunity to provide coordinated care and to adhere to quality metrics is in the wheelhouse of an EHR. All too often clinicians and practices shy away from utilizing new codes due to fear of being distracted or spending time and money for little additional reimbursement. *Suffice it to say, if a new code exists, it provides an opportunity to produce additional revenue.* That is the way that new codes must be approached. Granted, there are always risks that the cost and amount of time spent documenting for the new code will exceed the revenue that the code produces. With that said, it has been my experience that is usually not the case.

One of the best examples of this issue came to us at Senior Care of Colorado when the new PQRS system was put in place by Medicare. Documenting the PQRS codes might add 1–2 % of revenue per year, but the initial question that we had was whether the time our providers spent doing the work for these codes might easily reduce their productivity by more than 2 %. We actually ended up not coding PQRS during its first year for this reason. However, it became clear to us that there were opportunities to automate the process in a way that made it easier for our clinicians to document properly without diminishing their productivity. Furthermore, it also became clear that quality coding was not going away, and that over time, it would become ingrained in the coding system. Once you know what Medicare's plans are, you need to figure out how to implement processes internally to adhere to the new requirements!

23.5   Integrating Technologies in the Field

One of our greatest challenges in implementing our own EHR was what to do in the field. It was one thing to support the infrastructure to have computers in every exam room, but what could we do in nursing homes, or even during home visits? Early on, this presented a number of challenges, as our EHR wasn't easily accessed from outside. Again, these decisions required careful analysis of cost and benefit. If a provider productivity were to drop due to poor internet availability or a slow computer, that could be catastrophic. We actually approached this issue very slowly and carefully. It took several years and gradual piloting of approaches before we were able to get most of our physicians to utilize technology in the field. Fortunately, this issue is being solved to a greater degree every day with new software and new technology.

23.6 Technology and Productivity

There is a common thread, and that is the relationship between technology and productivity. In a fee-for-service world, this equation is linear. If the cost of technology (including the time to use it) exceeds any revenue gains related to productivity, there is a problem. This is always most simply looked at from the perspective of a reduction in productivity. One also has to be cautiously aware of the probability that the clinicians might be maintaining their productivity numbers at the cost of spending more hours in the day. This is not an uncommon reaction by healthcare providers, and sometimes only when they quit due to the impact of these added time demands will you be aware of the problem! It is critical for the practice to continually monitor their clinician's time as it relates to their productivity and to assess any dissatisfaction with the technology that you are utilizing.

The new world of reimbursement will reward outcomes and fee-for-service may not be the predominant mode of payment. What does that mean in regard to EHRs and productivity? New technology has the opportunity to enhance care coordination and reduce hospitalizations and overall healthcare expenditures. While it is possible that added time spent using technology will achieve a positive return on the investment, it still doesn't make sense to accept that as being okay. No matter the payment methodology, the more patients that an individual clinician can touch in a day, the better, with the caveat that the clinician must still spend the necessary amount of time to deliver upon the geriatric approach to care. If an hour with the patient and family is necessary, then so be it. However, if that hour becomes an hour and a half due to the technology and the same outcomes can be achieved in less time, then we should not be forgiving of the added time. I think that there has been too much acceptance of additional hassles caused by new technology. In my mind, this is unacceptable.

Future electronic health records should actually allow us to practice geriatrics the way we were trained and to coordinate that care effectively. It should not have us needlessly filling out forms or checking off unnecessary boxes. Until that day comes, however, we have to work with what we are given and figure out the most effective way of integrating it into our practices.

Opportunities in Today's Healthcare Marketplace

24

We are in the middle of a "Silver Tsunami" in the United States. The population is getting older and the demographic over 85 years of age is rapidly exploding. At the same time, the number of board-certified geriatricians is declining! There continue to be obstacles to the forces of traditional supply and demand principles. However, this should not distract us from the many opportunities in the healthcare marketplace for geriatricians and geriatric practices. In the midst of this fertile marketplace stands the belief among geriatricians and others that it is very difficult to succeed in the business of geriatrics. This book opened with a geriatric practice success story. I have tried to share many of the attributes that can be gleaned from such successes. There is ultimately only one way that we will determine if our confidence is well placed. *Health systems, practices, and clinicians alike must embrace the concept that geriatric practices can be profitable!*

One of my favorite techniques to approaching a business challenge is to understand the worst case scenario. I learned this method from Dr. Jim Riopelle during my years at GeriMed of America. To GeriMed, the failure of the Medicare program would be the ultimate worst case scenario. In regard to this possibility, we chose to take the premise that the government could not afford to fail when it comes to the healthcare needs of the elderly in this country. In many ways, this theory has held true since the founding of the Medicare program. Unfortunately, many of the methods that have been used to prop up the system have arguably harmed it. Nevertheless, there are lessons to be taken from the willingness of politicians from both sides of the aisle to constantly run their political campaigns with the promise "not to touch your Medicare!" Furthermore, if Medicare fails, there is a great likelihood that the entire healthcare system will fail as well. Worst case scenarios are not meant to be a deterrent to developing solutions to problems. They should actually be an incentive to figure out how to succeed. *We appear to be at a major tipping point in the development of the Medicare program, and it is critical that we determine effective solutions to the financial challenges faced by the program.*

© Springer International Publishing Switzerland 2016
M. Wasserman, *The Business of Geriatrics*, DOI 10.1007/978-3-319-28546-7_24

24.1 The Geriatric Approach to Care Finally Wins

I have spent a considerable amount of time in this book vouching for the value of the geriatric approach to care. Clearly, one must believe in that approach in order to move forward with any of the multiple opportunities that can and will exist for geriatricians and geriatric practices. It is critical that a practice must also support the execution of this principle with every fiber of its existence. *I believe that this is the single most important factor underlying successful approaches to improving the Medicare program.* Having recounted the challenges that geriatricians face throughout the pages of this book, it should be clear that optimism must be our friend if we are to succeed.

Geriatricians and geriatric practices should fully comprehend the value that their approach to care provides. They should be willing to share and advocate for the geriatric approach to care. Being tentative does no one any favors. Specialists of all ilk have no problem confidently promoting their approaches to care despite the fact that they rarely have any evidence supporting these approaches in older adults. It behooves us not only to be knowledgeable, but to be willing to share our successes in such a way as to demonstrate our confidence in the way we care for our patients. *That confidence is critical as opportunities to intercede are starting to occur all around us!*

24.2 Innovation Center Opportunities

The opportunities to provide a geriatric approach to care are occurring all over the United States. CMS's innovation program has seen to that. In fact, the first place that anyone should look in order to determine opportunities to develop a geriatric program or practice is at www.cms.gov. From there, it is easy to make a list of the myriad possibilities. CMS lists the following innovation models (www.innovation. cms.gov), some of which we have already discussed in this book:

- Accountable care
- Episode-based payment initiatives
- Primary care transformation
- Initiatives focused on Medicaid
- Initiative focused on Medicare-Medicaid enrollees
- Initiatives to accelerate the development and testing of new payment and service delivery models
- Initiatives to speed the adoption of best practices

Each of these innovation programs have maps that show where they are being carried out across the country. If you are willing to move anywhere, you might look for opportunities that best fit your interests and needs. If you already know where you want to practice, or have an existing practice in a particular locale, check out the maps and identify innovation projects in your area. If you are a physician practice management company, or a provider of healthcare services, you will ignore these opportunities at your own peril.

24.3   Identify the Opportunity

The first step is in identifying the opportunity. For example, you may find that a local hospital system has developed an accountable care organization or is participating in a bundled payment program. This is just the beginning. Just as starting a practice requires rigorous preparation, so does approaching one of these opportunities. It's important to do ones homework and to find out what's actually happening with a particular project in the community. Are the local physicians happy? Who is controlling the purse strings? Are there any other geriatricians already involved or potentially available to partner with? As we have recounted in previous chapters, it is important to identify the various ways that a geriatrician or geriatric practice can be of assistance. Is an ACE unit a viable option? Is there a need for a geriatric consultation service? How coordinated is the continuum of care?

Don't stop with the first identified opportunity. Look to see if there are others available in the community. They might be different programs, but you may find that they have similar needs. Where is there competition? Where is there no competition? Depending upon ones personal situation, might you consider moving to another area that has opportunities that fit your interests to a better degree? There are a multitude of programs going on right now, and very few of them have engaged geriatricians.

24.4   Seize the Moment!

You've identified the opportunity, now it's time to seize the moment! You've done your preparation. Now you need to get in front of the decision-makers. That may not be as difficult as you think. One of the fortunate aspects of having an M.D. after ones name is that people will meet with you. You certainly want to determine that you're meeting with the right person, but that can usually be found out with some very basic research. Once you've set up an appointment, you need to be prepared to sell yourself and the approach to care. In this circumstance, being a geriatrician and having credentials to match that are invaluable.

As we have stated many times throughout this book, one must be confident in their belief that the geriatric approach to care and model of care works. If you are not confident, you will never convince anyone else. Don't be afraid to share other's successful experiences. In fact, one of the reasons that I have shared real-life experiences in this book is so they can be utilized by others to promote the effectiveness of a geriatric practice. There is also some literature available in regard to programs like ACE, GRACE, and PACE. Use data whenever you can! Don't be afraid to use anecdotes. Many of the decision-makers that you will be speaking to have an older loved one who has suffered in our healthcare system. Take advantage of that!

Be specific about what you plan to do. This is your wheelhouse. They don't understand it. You need to tell them what they need and explain why they need it. Statistics can be very helpful in order to make your point, but won't always be readily available. However, there will be data demonstrating the significant costs and utilization by the frail elderly. The fact that you can impact those costs is a powerful incentive to consider a geriatric program. Remember, just because you can't guarantee outcomes should not be a reason not to make the case for what is possible. This is your area of expertise. This is your moment!

24.5   Execute the Geriatric Approach and Model

It's crunch time. You've made your case and the opportunity is now at hand. Getting up and running is arguably the most difficult aspect of any operation. Be honest with yourself about what is truly necessary for your practice to be successful. Do not cut corners when it comes to being able to provide quality care and service. Don't be afraid to ask for adequate resources and reimbursement. If you are taking an administrative or leadership role, make sure that you are paid fairly for the time you are putting in and the expertise that you are providing. *At the same time, it is critical that you make sure that the care you deliver is adequately compensated.*

If a portion of your practice is fee-for-service, make sure that you and your clinicians are well trained to appropriately code for the work that is done. If you are working in a capitated environment, do your homework and make sure that the amount you are receiving is adequate for the service you are providing. *Know your numbers!* The healthcare road is littered with great ideas that supposedly saved lots of money, but couldn't ultimately stand on their own two feet.

Stay true to the geriatric approach and model of care. This can be lost among other practical issues. It is the linchpin of your success. You must make sure that every clinician understands the geriatric approach. This is much harder than you might think. With a limited workforce of geriatricians and other healthcare professionals trained in geriatrics, it can be a challenge to identify and hire those who practice the geriatric approach to care. Ongoing education is a must. Reassurance is also necessary, as the outside healthcare world will often disparage the way that you care for patients. One of the great advantages of growing a large geriatric practice is the strength in numbers and the mutual support that a group of clinicians provide for one another. If we don't believe in what we do, we will not succeed. *The good news is that most geriatricians are quite passionate about how they care for patients!*

24.6   Promote Your Program and Accomplishments

Once you've put together a program and it is up and running, you cannot rest on your laurels. This can prove to be one of the most difficult things for geriatricians. As a group, clinicians who care for older adults tend to be more introverted.

Promoting what they do runs counter to their personality. Unfortunately, if you don't promote your program and what you've accomplished, others will take it for granted.

Promoting ones practice doesn't necessarily require boasting about it. Maintaining contact with other providers in the community is very important. Having relationships with the local home health companies is one example. Giving talks at the local senior center on successful aging can be a great way of getting the word out about your practice. Geriatric medicine is "motherhood and apple pie." People in the community will naturally appreciate what you do. They just need to know that you're doing it! One of my favorite lines is to tell people that I've discontinued more medications in my career than I've started. There aren't many physicians who can make this claim. Geriatricians generally can. People in the community love to hear this. In a world of rapidly rising pharmaceutical expenditures, health systems and insurers like to hear this as well.

Some of us live in a bubble. That bubble is made up of others who share our beliefs and approach to care. If we stay in that bubble, others will not be aware of what we can do. It's easy to feel like everything is working well within our own little world. Unfortunately, if others aren't aware of the type of care that we provide and the value in that care, we cannot expand. It is critical that all of us promote the type of care that we provide and how that care can benefit the older adults in our society.

24.7 Share Your Successes

While this book is written for the individual geriatrician and practice, there is a more global reality at stake. The future of geriatrics as a discipline may depend on our ability to share each and every one of our successes. Similarly, our individual success can be built upon our willingness to share our positive results and outcomes with those around us. This actually begins with the people who work for you. They need to know that the practice is achieving its goals. They also need to hear that the type of care they are used to delivering is being nurtured by the practice.

If you are the medical director of a nursing facility and you've helped the facility reduce its antipsychotic medication usage, make sure that the administrator is aware of how this has helped the facility's bottom line. If you have a contract with an insurer and you know that you are helping their profitability, make sure that they know about your results. Regular meetings with customers of the practice are important not only for maintaining relationships and identify problems, but to promote the positives.

We live in a healthcare world where a 20 % reduction in a particular outcome is touted, even when that decrease actually represents only one to two out of a hundred patients. It is ok to be proud of your individual successes and to share them as needed to allow you to achieve more of them. Don't forget to share your successes with yourself as well, you deserve it!

24.8   The Future Is Now!

This book opened with a story. It was a story based on a passion for the health and well-being of seniors in our country. Those of us in the field of geriatrics share this passion. That is without question. The problem is that many of us think it is either impossible or too difficult to make a geriatric practice financially viable. I hope that I have been able to dispel that belief. Just as we need to know the proper treatment for a chronic disease, businesses are no different. The principles and tools for success are available to us. The demographics are screaming for our services.

The healthcare marketplace is going through a whirlwind of changes. There are significant battles for control over how the healthcare dollar is spent. Hospitals are acquiring physician practices again. Physician practice management companies are getting involved in bundled payment models and accountable care organizations. Insurers are consolidating. While much of this creates challenges to the individual geriatrician, it also creates opportunities. The fact that the frail elderly are the highest utilizers of care is common knowledge. That puts us in a position to succeed. We just need to take hold of the ball and run with it.

Index

© Springer International Publishing Switzerland 2016
M. Wasserman, *The Business of Geriatrics*, DOI 10.1007/978-3-319-28546-7

Printed in the United States
By Bookmasters